VODOU SAINTS
Lessons on Life, Death and Resurrection From Haiti

Arthur M. Fournier, M.D.

Oct. 13, 2012

David and Suzy —

Enjoy the story!

Art

Published by

B&B
Press

For information, go to www.booksandbooks.com

Published by B & B Press
Mitchell@booksandbooks.com

A Motherland Production

Creative: Petra Mason

Designed by Cindy Seip
www.splashfoto.com

Library of Congress Cataloging-in-Publication Date
Vodou Saints / by Arthur M. Fournier, M.D.

For information about special discounts for bulk purchases,
please contact www.booksandbooks.com

Library of Congress Control Number: 2012947198

First Edition
1 2 3 4 5 6 7 8 9 10

ISBN: 978-0-9839378-5-2

Dedication

To the victims of the AIDS epidemic, particularly Regis -
Nou pap bliye'w - We'll not forget you

To Janet –
My reluctant Mary/Athena/Erzilie/Earth Mother/Vodou Saint
You'll always be with us.

To the victims of the January 12th earthquake -
Nou toujou ak nou - You are always with us.
To the survivors of the quake -
Kenbe fem - Stay the course.

VODOU SAINTS

Contents

VODOU SAINTS

About the Title

Vodou Saints is the English transliteration of the Kreyol word *Vodouisant*. You'll find true *Vodouisants* in this book, from the Haitians persecuted for having AIDS, to the courageous survivors of Haiti's infamous earthquake. For Haitians, the word is shorthand for the unique Haitian worldview, for which Vodou is an integral part. There are other Vodou Saints captured in these pages also – the idea of Vodou Saints started as a metaphor for people who aspired to a virtuous life, even if they did not adhere to a formal religion. As the story unfolded, however the metaphor evolved also, to include all those, Haitians and non-Haitians, who search for meaning in everything – a principle tenet of Vodou, and all those who came forward to help and learn from Haitians in the country's hour of greatest need.

About the Cover:
A portrait of Erzilie, in the style of Saintilus Ismael, painted by an unknown street artist.

VODOU SAINTS

Preface

Vodou Saints is a memoir in three parts focusing on lessons I have learned from Haiti and its people.

Part 1, Destiny's Child begins the story of the earthquake of January 12th, 2010 and how it affected my life as a doctor and a person, particularly in the extraordinary chain of events that lead to the rescue of the Baby Jenny.

Part II, Secrets of the Zombie Curse, chronicles the stigmatization of Haitian-Americans in Miami during the early days of the AIDS epidemic and what I learned from Haitians about the root causes of this modern plague. Those lessons on life and death took on deeper, personal meaning when my wife succumbed to Lou Gehrig's disease in 2007.

Part III, Lespwa Fe Viv, deals with lessons of life and death on a much grander scale--how the resilience, fortitude and spirituality of Haiti's people emerged in the wake of the earthquake; how a country came back from the brink of death.

Part I
Destiny's Child

1

A Prayer that is Sung is Twice the Prayer

Nadine struggled to her feet, but the shaking threw her once again to the floor. She rose to cross the living room of her family's fifth floor apartment struggling to reach the bedroom where her infant daughter Jenny and her babysitter, Marie Ange, were trapped. Just prior to the violent shaking Nadine would later learn was an earthquake, Marie Ange was singing a lullaby to Jenny, as she drifted off to sleep for a nap. Nadine's husband, Junior, was out interviewing for a singing job at a local nightclub. Nadine, just returned from a doctor's visit and visit to the pharmacy, had been preparing supper in the kitchen. As the floor wobbled underneath her feet, Nadine stumbled toward the door and went sprawling again. She could not see behind the closed door of the bedroom where Marie-Ange, a thirty something woman, lay on the floor, covering the infant from the plaster and concrete already falling from the ceiling. It was January 12, 2010 at 5:24 pm.

Haiti's earthquake did not give its victims any warning in the form of a preliminary trembler or a growing crescendo of noise. No, it started in full-intensity from its first instant – a violent roar of upheaval lasting thirty five seconds. The fifth floor of Nadine's apartment overlooking Rue Canapé Vert in Port au Prince filled with the roar of what sounded like a thousand pile-drivers smashing rock. Nadine rose again and stumbled toward the door. Suddenly, like the trap door of a gallows, the floor gave way and Nadine plunged into a vortex of collapsing walls, plaster, and concrete, screaming her baby's name as she fell.

Nadine's landing knocked the wind out of her and falling chunks of ceiling knocked her unconscious. Debris from her now destroyed apartment landed on top of her and buried her. Dust and aerosolized concrete choked her breathing. Immersed in total darkness and pinned, she was almost crushed by the weight of debris above her. As the hours passed after the quake, Nadine lapsed in and out of consciousness. She had no idea of what happened. In spite of her confusion, she thought of Jenny. Haitians believe that a prayer that's sung is twice the prayer. In spite of the dust that was choking her and the darkness and debris that entombed her, Nadine willed a hymn from her lungs and her heart – a hymn to Erzilie, the protectress of all things maternal. *"Tanpri, Erzilie,"* (please Erzilie), *sove bebe mwen* (save my child)."

In the rubble nearby Marie Ange was dead. We don't know exactly what killed Jenny's babysitter-- a blow to the head, a broken neck or the crushing weight of debris on top of her. Nor do we know how long she clung to life after the quake. We do know that Marie-Ange curled herself in a ball as the floor gave way, doing all she could to protect the infant in her arms. And as she lay dying, she did what she could to protect the child in whose care she had been entrusted. In this regard, she was only partially successful- some piece of debris had fractured Jenny's skull. Either the weight of Marie-Ange's body or the pile of rubble on top of them had also broken several of her ribs, on each side of her sternum. But her embrace was a key to Jenny's survival – when Jenny was found five days later, she was still wrapped in Marie-Ange's arms.

2

Baron Samedi's Greatest Hits

I was driving north on N.W. 7th Avenue in Miami. I had left my office at The University of Miami/Jackson Memorial Hospital Medical Center, heading for my condo in Aventura. Vigilant in avoiding Miami's rush hour kamikaze drivers, I did not care to be distracted by the ringing of my cell phone. It was Larry Pierre – a physician with whom I had collaborated in establishing a medical clinic in Miami's Little Haiti neighborhood. Larry, who had been the first Haitian-American doctor in Miami willing to confront the AIDS epidemic, is a man driven to serve his community. Since usually his calls concerned politics, I couldn't imagine why he needed to talk during rush hour. I was about to ask if this couldn't this wait until morning.

"There's been an earthquake in Haiti," he whispered, almost as if sharing a secret. "Have you heard?"

"No…" I faltered, suddenly hoping this news would prove to one of those baseless or exaggerated rumors that circulate in the Haitian diaspora of south Florida at Internet speed.

"It's going to be bad," Larry intoned. "I'll keep you posted…"

My ride home was then punctuated by a string of calls. I heard from our Haitian-American faculty at the University of Miami where I have worked for the past thirty-two years. I heard from friends of Project Medishare, a nonprofit public health organization for Haiti that I founded with Dr. Barth Green in 1994. I talked to Barth and to Ellen Powers, the Executive Director for Medishare. We all tried to milk each other for more information – we knew something very bad had happened. For me this was more than a medical emergency to be handled professionally. Over the decades, Haiti and its people had become a major part of my life, first through my Haitian-American patients with AIDS and then through my public health work in the Haitian countryside. In sixteen years, I had taken one hundred and seventeen trips to the island. In many ways, the Haitian worldview had become my own.

When I got home, I found an email from Barth.

"I'm heading down to Port au Prince tomorrow morning," he wrote. "I've got a private plane donated and clearance from Southcom. R u in?"

It was typical of Barth to take decisive action while the rest of us were still grappling with the bad news. He and I are like ying and yang. He's the quintessential surgical specialist. I'm a generalist, a family doctor. He is focused and driven, a man of action. I tended to be more contemplative.

"Can't," I typed. "I've got a root canal scheduled for Thursday afternoon and a 'Thank You Dinner' with Alonzo Mourning Thursday evening. Who'd you get the plane from? Don't you think we ought to at least wait to find out if the runaway is intact?"

Barth, as frequently happened, was a couple steps ahead of me. He wrote that Ken Ascher, a local philanthropist had donated his own plane and that they had already checked out the integrity of the runway, through contacts at the Southern Command (SouthCom).

"It's fine," Barth said. "I need to see the situation on the ground."

"How long do we have the plane for?" I asked.

"As long as we need it," he said. But if you're staying behind, I'll send you some phone numbers of others I know with planes – we'll need more!"

"O.K.," I replied. "I'll come down Friday with reinforcements."

Not until the following morning did we learn how terrible the earthquake really was. CNN reported "massive destruction" from a quake measuring 7.2 on the Richter scale, with an epicenter 6 miles southwest of Port au Prince. Lights and communications were down throughout the city.

At the office, Dr. Michel Dodard was the first of my Haitian-American colleagues to arrive. He was ashen and trembling.

"You better sit down" he said, and then took his own advice. Committed to Medishare from its inception, Michel is a thoughtful man with a vast knowledge of all things Haitian.

"I spoke with my brothers via Skype," he said. "All the Digicel towers are down, so forget trying to reach someone via cell phone. They and their families are fine, Merci à Dieu, but prepare yourself--all of Port au Prince is gone. Philippe can see its remains from the terrace of his home in Montagne Noire. It's a pile of rubble. Even the National Cathedral is down. Pétionville is not much better. All the roads are blocked by debris – everyone is a prisoner in their own home... I heard Barth is on his way down in a private plane. I hope he'll be able to land."

"Yes – he e-mailed me last night," I said. "I tried to talk him out of it, but you know Barth."

As the day progressed, more news filtered in, primarily via *teledyol* (word of mouth). Most of the families of our Haitian-American faculty survived, although some were injured. The families of our nurses and hospital staff did not fare as well. Part of the General Hospital, the main hospital for the poor in Port au Prince had collapsed, as had a hospital in Pétionville. The medical school was severely damaged. The control tower at the airport was shattered, although there was some hope the tarmac had escaped undamaged. The Episcopal Cathedral, with its historic murals depicting the life of Jesus, joined its Catholic counterpart on the list of the fallen. There were reports that the Hotel Montana, a favorite haven of visiting dignitaries, had collapsed, trapping the U.N. command inside. No word, however, on Hotel Villa Creole where Project Medishare volunteers usually stayed when in Port au Prince.

There was some small good news from Thomonde. This town, located on the Haiti's central plateau, sixty miles northeast of the capital, is home to Project Medishare's biggest operations, including a sixteen-bed hospital, a clinic, and administrative center for community health projects throughout surrounding communities. The quake was felt in Thomonde but caused little damage. Marie, a Haitian-American nurse who moved from Miami to Thomonde to run the Medishare operations was unhurt, as was our staff and a small team of nursing students visiting from University of Miami. Marie did not know if her apartment in Port au Prince survived. She was also distraught over the fact she could not communicate with her cook and housekeeper. She assumed that they had perished.

That night the first few photos of the devastation appeared on the news. They didn't look so awful. Based on the reports we had received, however, we knew that appearances were deceiving. These pictures, sent by survivors via cell phone from the less damaged parts of the city, conveyed false hope. Eyewitness accounts spoke of total devastation, streets blocked by rubble and dead bodies, survivors clawing with their bare hands, trying to extract loved ones from the wreckage.

Haitians find meaning in everything. It's a central tenet of Vodou, the country's shared faith that combines West African and Catholic rituals, traditions and values. Events in the world have particular meaning. There is, however, no guarantee that *Vodouisants,* as believers are known, will agree on what that meaning is. Speculation on the metaphysical significance of the earthquake began immediately, on both sides of the Windward Passage. Some, mostly members of Protestant denominations who equate Vodou with devil worship, sided with the American televangelist, Pat Robertson, who told CNN about the old myth that God placed a curse on Haitians as a result of their ancestors' pact with the devil to drive out the French slave regime in 1804. There was a grain of truth in Robertson's pontifications: The slaves who revolted refused to accept the French God and refused to give up their African identity. Vodou and the African values it represented were the heart of the world's only successful slave rebellion. Otherwise, Robertson was merely echoing the racist idea that the black men could not defeat godly white men without the treacherous help of Satan.

Vodouisants saw the epic disaster in a different light than Pastor Robertson -- in fact, as a rainbow of various hues. Perhaps the earthquake was the ultimate trick of Baron Samedi, the Vodou trickster who harvests the souls of the dead and escorts them to Paradise. Baron Samedi, like Pluto in Roman mythology or Vulcan in Greek, is a capricious god who comes and goes from the underworld. Alternatively, perhaps Bondye, the ultimate deity of Voudou, was actually being merciful, granting those who died an instant death and quick passage to the paradise of Guinea. For survivors, perhaps the quake and its aftermath was just one more mountain in the endless stream of mountains that Vodouisants must endure as the price of their freedom.

I also tried to find meaning in all this. Maybe, just maybe, Haiti's turbulent past would die with the earthquake's victims, and that a new Haiti would be born. Perhaps the self-discipline and motivation to lead a good life helping others, purely because it's the right thing to do, so central to Vodou, would finally prevail over the cynical realpolitik that has long dominated the Haitian capital of Port au Prince. Haitians would have to decide.

3
The Singer

Junior Alexis was walking Rue Canapé Vert in Port au Prince when the earthquake struck. He was returning from a job interview at a nearby club where he applied for a singing job. Junior is about thirty years old, a popular music performer known around Port au Prince. As he hiked up the hill, he was anticipating his nightly reunion with Nadine, his wife of a year and half, and their eight week old daughter. He passed the doors and windows of doctors' and lawyers' offices. He passed restaurants and clinics, a college, and couple of private schools. Rue Canapé Vert was a microcosm of all the changes that had afflicted Port au Prince over the last half-century. Originally a major thoroughfare, it linked the port, ministries, and commercial districts of Port au Prince with the comfortable homes of the elite and professional class halfway up in the mountain in Petionville, the capital's most affluent suburb. Over the years, the ravine and the hills surrounding the road had grown thick with *"bidonville"* (squatter's settlements) – flimsy homes built one cinderblock at a time by impoverished Haitians moving in from the countryside. The sidewalks were now swollen with street vendors selling produce, used clothes, chickens, goats, and shoes.

When the earthquake struck, Junior fell prostrate with the first jolt, covering his head with his right arm while trying to anchor himself to the sidewalk with the fingernails of his left hand. When the roaring and shaking stopped, he lifted his head and opened his eyes. A totally alien landscape confronted him.

The schools and stores that lined the Rue Canapé Vert were all flattened like crepes. The *bidonvilles* had slid down the hillside, filing the ravine with rubble. A cloud of dust stung his eyes and skin, blurring the shadows in the fading light and worsening his disorientation. To find Nadine, he knew he had to go up the hill and to the left. He stumbled forward at first, climbing over piles of crumbled concrete that blocked his way. Horns blared, as cars futilely attempted to ascend the route. Survivors with mangled limbs clawed their way out of doorways. Children screamed in pain. Some survivors called out for loved ones, while others called for help or wandered aimlessly in shock amidst the moans of the dying. Junior broke into a run, in spite of his trouble breathing and the cloud of dust that obscured all landmarks.

His neighborhood was now a moonscape of collapsed buildings. Recognizing the roof of the house that had once stood next door to his own, Junior identified the pile of concrete that used to be his home. He leapt on to a crumbled slab of roof and began heaving off blocks of debris, digging through the concrete powder and dust that clogged every crevice. Shards of concrete and splinters of wood cut his fingers as he dug. He had to find Nadine and

Jenny. The light was dying and soon there would be total darkness.

His calls of "Nadine! Nadine!" were greeted by silence. It had been a difficult pregnancy and labor for Nadine. At one point, the doctors had even told them it was quite possible that neither mother nor baby would survive childbirth. Nadine's labor finally ended with a healthy baby, but left her exhausted. As soon as Nadine returned home from the hospital, Junior had hired Marie-Ange to help care for the baby and Nadine. By Port au Prince standards, Nadine and Junior had a reasonably comfortable life with Junior making a decent living, mostly on tips, for his singing appearances.

Junior stopped at the sight of the bodies of two cousins who lived on the floors below them in their five-story apartment building. There was no time to mourn. He pulled their corpses from the wreckage, straightened out their bodies on the sidewalk, and folded their arms across their chest to give them a modicum of decency in death. Then, as quickly as he could, he re-entered the tunnel he had begun to dig into the rubble of his former apartment building.

The structure had not so much collapsed as imploded. On the outside, it looked like a ruined Egyptian pyramid, but as he broke through the outer shell of rubble he discovered crawl spaces and lean-tos formed by partially preserved but shattered walls and ceilings, almost like a house of cards. Then, through the sound of concrete and sand settling through the empty spaces, he heard a cough, and then another and then a groan. It was Nadine, wedged in a small triangular space just ahead. She was covered in dust, had a gash on her forehead and abrasions on her face. She was unconscious, but breathing, grimacing and making feeble movements with her arms and legs.

Junior first widened the tunnel that led him in. It took all his strength to extract his wife from the rubble. Once he had dragged her outside, he went in again to look for Jenny. There was no sign of her. When he returned to Nadine, she could not answer his questions as to Jenny's whereabouts. A decision had to be made. With little light left, further digging for Jenny would be futile, and who knew how serious Nadine's injuries might be? He called over some youths and pleaded for their help. Together he and these young men picked up Nadine and carried her down the hill to Hôpital Canapé Vert.

Prior to the quake, Hôpital Canapé Vert was the preferred hospital for Port au Prince's elite. Now it was partially collapsed, the medical and nursing staff nowhere to be seen. There were, however, abandoned cars in the parking lot. Junior settled Nadine into the back seat of one of these cars, then, exhausted, slipped into a troubled sleep. Maybe a doctor would show up by daylight.

The next day, a doctor, did indeed, come. Junior accosted him and asked him to examine Nadine. His report was reassuring. Nadine was suffering from a concussion, but had no broken bones or serious injuries. The doctor expected her to make a full recovery. Junior looked skyward and thanked Bondye. At least one of his prayers had been answered. He decided to keep vigil with Nadine for the rest of that day.

As for Jenny, he would return to look for at first light the next day.

4
Music

Romel Joseph was on the third floor of his music school when the earthquake struck, practicing his violin. His pregnant wife, Myslie, on the first floor, was crushed and instantly killed. Romel fell three stories and was immediately pummeled by debris from above. Concrete blocks crushed both his legs. Another block broke three fingers in his left hand – the critical hand that a concert violinist needs to finger his notes.

If ever there were an example of the indomitable spirit so many Haitians manifest, Romel was it. He was born to a poor Haitian family in the small rural town of Gros Morne. Blinded at birth by an infection, his parents sent him to a school for the handicapped in Port au Prince.

Romel turned out to be a prodigy – mastering both the violin and piano while still a child. His talent earned him scholarships – first to the University of Cincinnati School of Music and then the Julliard School.

As a world-renowned concert violinist, his performances commanded considerable compensation, but he never forgot his humble roots. He plowed his earnings into his music school in Haiti – a school specifically where poor children could learn music. When the school burned down (ironically, in January 12, 2000 – exactly ten years before the quake) he rebuilt it. At the time of the quake he had 300 children enrolled. Fortunately, they had all returned to their homes for the evening when the quake struck.

Any movement by Romel provoked excruciating pain, so he lay motionless in the cramped space he later termed "my coffin." To keep his sanity and distract himself from his pain, he played in his mind his entire repertoire. That filled the eighteen hours until his students returned the following day to free him.

The doctors who examined him after he was extracted from the rubble told him he would die if he stayed in Haiti – gangrene would assuredly infect his leg wounds. They also told him that he would never play the violin again. Romel, however, was not about to let Baron Samedi ruin his plans for his music school. In fact, he had a trump card to play against the trickster – during his time at school in the United State he became a U.S. citizen. He went to the embassy in a wheelchair and showed his passport. He was air-evacuated later that afternoon to Miami and admitted directly to the trauma service at Jackson Memorial Hospital, where the doctors set his broken bones and debrided his wounds. Three pins aligned the bones that were shattered in his left hand. "There's hope you can play again," his doctor told him, "although I'm making no promises…"

Hope. *Lespwa.* Music to Romel's ears

5
Into the Inferno

True to his credo of "lead, follow or get out of the way," Barth Green arrived in Port au Prince, along with two trauma surgeons he had cajoled into accompanying him. He found the airport abandoned and Port au Prince descending into anarchy. He made his way to the nearby compound of the United Nations. The U.N. has stationed a peacekeeping force in Haiti since 1994 which focused solely on security. After the earthquake, the Haitian government was paralyzed, leaving the U.N. as the only functioning authority in the country. As the sole organization with manpower, machinery, and supplies available to respond, the U.N. reluctantly took on a disaster-relief role. By the time Barth arrived, U.N. workers had already brought in over two hundred critically injured patients stacked in cots under two open-air tents. The dead were stored in a metal container, located between the two tents, which served as a makeshift morgue.

Barth struck a bargain with the U.N. commander: let volunteers stay in the U.N. compound and Medishare would turn the two tents into a field hospital to treat victims of the quake. Barth texted this news to me and other Project Medishare faculty in Miami. He also gave us our marching orders – get more planes, equipment, and supplies. The horror of what happened began to sink in.

"It's hell here!" he wrote, tersely. "We lost our Port au Prince head-quarters in Paco and Marie believes her cook and housekeeper were killed. We need ketamine for anesthesia. Have done lots of amputations without and it's not very humane! Thank you. The stench of death is everywhere. Send large black plastic bags so that we can dispose have amputated body parts. Lots of them!"

The two tents, he reported, each held about a hundred severely injured patients, lying in stretchers, many with family members attending to their needs. The tents were dubbed "The MINUSTAH Surgical Hospital." MINUSTAH is the French acronym for the U.N. mission in Haiti. The name was a bit of an exaggeration, since it was impossible to perform all but the most brutal surgery without operating rooms and anesthesia. The "hospital" lacked water, food, toilets, or quarters for volunteer staff.

The donated plane returned to Miami to pick up another trauma surgeon, some volunteer orthopedic and surgical residents, as well as surgical supplies, I.V.'s, and antibiotics and took off for Port au Prince. Also on the plane were some news reporters looking to get quickly to the scene of an epic story. In fact, I spent a sizable portion of my time after the quake, before I left for Haiti, talking with producers and editors desperate to get their crews into the disaster zone. Medishare agreed to take several media crews, including Elizabeth Cohen from CNN and Jennifer Ashton of CBS. As a bargaining chip, the CBS producer reminded us that Jennifer was a doctor – a practicing obstetrician/gynecologist who would also see patients when she wasn't reporting.

I cancelled my root canal for Thursday afternoon. I would need my unanesthetized mouth to speak that evening with Alonzo Mourning, the retired all-star basketball player for the Miami Heat, who supports a youth center in Overtown, one of Miami's historically black neighborhoods. I had met Alonzo in 2008 when he asked the University of Miami medical school to set up a health room at the center. The task was assigned to my office, and we delivered the goods. In return, for two years in a row, I was invited to an annual "Thank You Dinner" Alonzo organized for all the contributors to the Overtown Youth Center. Alonzo impressed me as a humble person who was devoted to children from disadvantaged backgrounds. I privately hoped that someday I might get him down to Haiti to see our work there but wanted to earn some credibility with him first through our work at the Youth Center.

The second annual "Thank You Dinner" took place two days after the earthquake. It was well attended by Miami's philanthropists, power attorneys, public-minded businessmen, and others. Alonzo and a small group were listening, as I spoke about the problems we were finding among the children of Overtown Youth Center, particularly in the realm of mental health. I talked about the failure of Medicaid to meet their needs and the importance of providing dental services. Then Alonzo asked me about Haiti.

"Dr. Green is already down there," I said. "He says its hell on Earth. I'm going down tomorrow morning--on Eric's plane, I might add." Eric Feder, a businessman, sitting next to Alonzo had called me earlier in the day to say he was putting his private planes at the disposal of Medishare. I looked to Alonzo.

"Do you want to come?"

He thought for about five seconds.

"Yes, I would."

Saving the life of baby Jenny would require a very skilled team. On day two after the quake, that team was converging on Port au Prince.

Dr. Karen Schneider, a pediatrician who worked at Johns Hopkins Hospital in Baltimore, was already on her way down to Haiti when the earthquake struck. She had volunteered to work at an orphanage there for several years before the quake. This was supposed to be a routine mission. Now she found herself marooned by the quake in the Fort Lauderdale airport. Fortunately, she had friends in Miami who told her of Project Medishare. She called our "command center" and volunteered. She was on our third flight down on the second day.

Karen Chamuel was a recently graduated nurse practitioner who had previously worked in Jackson Memorial Hospital's Pediatric Intensive Care Unit. The images from Haiti that started to trickle in from the media had moved her to tears. She asked her supervisor for leave, which was immediately granted. She had the foresight to fill her duffel bag with what she anticipated would be much needed supplies – gauze pads, gloves, and stuff to start I.V.'s. She also arrived on the third flight after the quake. All that night she and the other Karen, the pediatrician, examined, evaluated and tended to the wounds of the approximately 75 children already in our care.

The first plane from Miami on the third day after the earthquake was a twelve seat Gulfstream jet that departed from Opa-Locka Airport. Other volunteers on that flight, beside myself, included a Haitian-American surgeon, his son, a Haitian-American physician, several Haitian-American and American nurses and Dave, a faculty-physician from UM's Department of Orthopedics.

This, my 118th trip to Haiti, would be like no other. All previous trips had been on commercial airlines. Given the situation we were flying down into in Haiti, the casualness of the waiting area, the simplicity of security clearance and the plushness of the private plane were guilty pleasures. In fact, none of us had ever traveled in such luxury – the wide, pivoting leather seats, wood paneling, high-definition television and wet-bar would, in retrospect, stand in stark contrast to the spartan conditions that awaited us.

Alonzo arrived fifteen minutes before our scheduled departure, with no entourage, carrying a Miami Heat duffle bag. I had warned the other passengers in advance that we might have a "special guest." Even with that heads-up, eyes widened and jaws dropped when he entered. At six feet ten inches tall, his physical presence commands attention.

The flight to Port au Prince took only an hour and a half. Most non-Haitians from Miami know little about Haiti and what they do know they derive from a media filter that often focuses on the abject poverty, political in-fighting and violence of the capital. Such a focus provides a narrow and biased view of Haiti, at least in the opinion of Haitians and those Americans, like myself, who've grown to love its people. The Haitian-Americans on the team, with a little prodding from me, took the opportunity to tell the new-comers to Haiti, including Alonzo, the fuller story of Haiti. The only country in the world created by a slave revolt, the second modern republic in the world after the United States, and the first black republic, whose historic ostracism preserved its unique African culture, language, and worldview. Alonzo listened intently.

Because of the high volume of relief planes, we were forced to circle the capital several times before landing. It was a clear morning and as I stared out the window, the magnitude of the tragedy below became all too apparent. The city I had flown into so often – the city I had taken for granted would always be there – was, for the most part, gone, – replaced by a gray-brown landscape of concrete rubble, dust and dirt.

After we finally landed, our jet taxied into a space in front of the terminal. On our left were two large airbuses – one from Canada and one with Hebrew lettering, which I assumed was from Israel. On our right were several C-130's and helicopters. As we stepped on to the tarmac I noted several large, distinct crowds milling about. Off in the distance, troops in camouflage gathered en masse, as well as several groups of fire-rescue teams, all in different colored uniforms. Another group was sitting quietly in the shade of the abandoned terminal, with suitcases and other luggage - most likely U.S. citizens waiting to be evacuated. Closer to us, workers bustled about, moving palettes of supplies with forklifts.

We were greeted by Marie, Medishare's director in Thomonde, and

Pasha and Angel, volunteers from a prominent Haitian family who offered to handle the logistics of our teams. They had a large van and several trucks to transport people and bags to the Project Medishare tents, along with our cargo of precious antibiotics and even more precious morphine. I talked briefly with fire–rescue teams from Boston (my hometown) and Miami, and explored the inside of the airport – moving freely through areas normally restricted to access. The damage in the terminal was not as severe as we had heard - reports of the control tower's collapse were greatly exaggerated. The windows had been shattered and the sprinklers system had been accidentally activated. Puddles of water and sodden ceiling tiles littered the floor. A flabbergasted reporter from ABC noticed Alonzo and tried to interview him. He refused, however, saying only "I just arrived," and, "I'm just here to see this with my own eyes." Soon, a U.N. escort would lead us through checkpoints and into the bowels of the U.N. compound.

As I scanned the crowd of reporters, I made eye contact with a familiar face. It was Kathie Klarreich. Our paths had crossed only once before – we both served on a panel discussion about Haiti - but I knew her as a fellow writer about Haiti. Originally from Ohio, life's twists and turns brought her to Haiti about twenty years ago. Like me, she developed a deep affection for the Haitian people – a story she tells in her memoir, "Madame Dread."

"What are you doing here?" I asked, as we hugged and kissed on both cheeks, Haitian-style.

"Free-lancing" she answered casually as she looked past me to Alonzo.

"I hear you've got quite an operation going on in the U.N. compound. There's not much happening here. Mind if I tag along?"

6
Controlled Chaos

On the third day, the U.S. Army had arrived in force. After it secured the airport and established air traffic control, the airport was transformed into Port au Prince's lifeline, with military, fire-rescue, and international forces arriving around the clock. Departing planes began evacuating the estimated twenty thousand American citizens stranded in Haiti. By State Department decree, however, no Haitians were allowed to leave, no matter how critically injured. This created a humanitarian dilemma for relief workers, as there were no functioning Haitian facilities with the capacity to care for the thousands of patients with broken bones and crush injuries being brought in to the makeshift first-aid stations and clinics springing up throughout the city. To paper over this problem, the UN negotiated a small number of emergency evacuations (fifteen at most) each day to the Dominican Republic and Martinique.

Project Medishare was one of the few non-governmental organizations bringing in volunteers to any significant degree. In fact, thanks in large part to Barth, three private planes a day were making round-trips between South Florida and Port au Prince, carrying doctors, nurses, Kreyol translators, and medical supplies in bulk quantities. The Medishare hospital's location in close proximity to the airport and relative abundance of doctors, medicines and supplies soon made it a magnet for the most severely injured, in spite of the primitive conditions.

New volunteers were oriented upon arrival by Dr. Enrique Ginzburg, the trauma surgeon who accompanied Barth the morning after the quake. After three days of non-stop work, Enrique had somewhat the appearance of a mad scientist. Dressed in a soiled and sweat-stained scrub top and jeans, his hair was unkempt and his beard untrimmed. His eyes had the sort of stare seen in hyperthyroidism or extreme fright – the effect of the adrenaline rush necessary to function in crisis mode for three days without sleep.

"Make sure you all sign in" he reminded the new arrivals, "and don't leave the compound."

He then separated the group into doctors and nurses and asked everyone to identify themselves and their specialty. New arrivals would be paired with "veterans" who had arrived earlier. There would be two twelve-hour shifts for two teams, each with two team leaders.

"Try to make sure each team has at least one Kreyol speaker" he advised.

There were no toilets, he warned us. Volunteers should sleep on the platform or in chairs in front of the first tent. He hoped they had received the message about bringing their own supplies – they were on their own with regard to food and water.

Within minutes the new arrivals had integrated themselves into the existing teams. Their patients had no charts - just notes on scraps of paper taped to their bedclothes. Boys, girls, men, and women were randomly scattered on cots between the two tents. I.V.'s were suspended from a spider web of clotheslines woven at eye-level through both tents. Injuries were diagnosed by physical examination alone and they were gruesome: broken limbs, crushed pelvises, smashed faces. Traditional lines of authority between doctors and nurses were blurred – it was the team's responsibility to see that I.V.'s didn't run out, that dressings were changed and that morphine and antibiotics were given on time.

While the volunteers began their work, Enrique took the reporters on a tour, starting outside the tent at a table.

"This is our operating   room," he declared. "We need the sunlight to see the pumpers [surgical jargon for bleeding arteries]. Lots of amputations – we first try to set the bones and give antibiotics, but if they get gangrene, the limb's got to go. It's Gettysburg medicine…"

Returning inside the tent, the reporters witnessed scenes that would shock even the most hardened combat veterans. Many patients were still covered in concrete dust, giving their countenances a ghost-like appearance. The bloodstains on their clothes, made them look like ghouls from a horror movie. Many were unconscious, some sweating with fever, most moaning, and writhing in pain. The first batch of morphine had just arrived on our plane that morning, and there had not yet been time to administer it. A fetid odor – a mixture of the scents of sweat, pus, urine, and feces – permeated the tents.

Dave, the orthopedic surgeon who flew in with me on the morning plane was soon in high gear. Assisted by an orthopedic resident who had flown in earlier, he quickly moved from stretcher to stretcher, checking wounds, changing dressings, splinting fractures with layers of cardboard strips cut from boxes. Alonzo worked as a nurse, holding up limbs while Dave wrapped them in gauze, carrying patients with his bare arms to and from the operating table, and picking up trash.

The following morning, things had improved in the field hospital. Patients' families and night shift volunteers had bathed all of the patients, using bottled water flown in on the previous night's flight. The odor of bodily fluids, so pungent the night before, was now tolerable. Morphine and the makeshift splints that Dave and the orthopedic residents had applied during the might went a long way towards relieving the suffering of our patients. In the early morning light, most were sleeping, although some were talking with family members or praying. The one exception was an unfortunate woman in the forward tent who the night shift dubbed "the singer." She suffered from a crushed pelvis. No amount of morphine could relieve her pain, so she coped by continuously singing and praying. When exhaustion overcame her, she would lapse into a fitful sleep for a few minutes, then awake in pain, and start singing again.

Come morning, a miracle akin to the biblical miracle of the loaves and fishes delivered a small breakfast to all patients. Some of the food was brought in by family members, some provided by the volunteers who ate granola bars and drank bottled water. After breakfast, the teams rounded through the tents, identifying those patients who were improving, those in need of emergency surgery, and those who might need to be transferred to the Dominican Republic or Martinique.

More patients had improved than had deteriorated. Only one patient expired the night before, down from ten the previous day. Most patients who were conscious smiled and thanked us as we checked their injuries. Enrique identified four patients who had developed gangrene or infections severe enough to warrant emergency amputations. Others would require dressing changes - a painful procedure under these circumstances – or replacing their splints with casts. The first rolls of plaster and casting supplies were expected to arrive on the next flight. Almost every patient needed a lot of I.V. fluids to keep their kidneys from shutting down, so the I.V. bags needed constant monitoring and frequent changing.

In the United States there's a certain dynamic tension between physicians and surgeons – they are trained differently, they think differently and have different skill sets. There's also a hierarchal relationship between doctors and nurses that simmers with the stress of critically ill patients and occasionally boils over. Worst, though, is the persuasive attitude that our patients have become the enemy. This attitude starts during the dehumanizing process of residency training in medical school and esca-lates in practice, where the need to see volumes of patients in order to make a living, coupled with fear of lawsuits, has created an environment in which doctors, nurses and patients are all suspicious of one another.

Not here. In one day, all of us--physicians, surgeons, nurses, students, patients, and a retired professional basketball player – had become a band of brothers and sisters. Dave, the orthopod, his scrubs drenched with sweat, exclaimed, "I'm loving it!" when asked how he was holding up. He refused to be relieved at the end of the day shift, as he eagerly awaited the arrival of plaster.

"This is what I went to medical school for," Enrique said, as he and Alonzo lifted a patient out of her cot and on to our makeshift operating table. "Not the b.s. I have to put up with back home."

For me, it was a scene pregnant with irony. I had become disillu-sioned with my profession back home – our enslavement by technology, our treatment of patients as consumers, healthcare as a commodity, and particularly, its impotency in relieving my wife Janet's suffering in the last year of her life. Haiti helped me rediscover my moral compass. In these most squalid of conditions, my colleagues were rediscovering that impulse to just help our fellow man. "Too bad it took hundreds of thousands of dead and injured to wake them up," I mused "and don't dwell on how long it will take to lapse into their old ways when they return home." Still, hope makes us live, and perhaps there was hope that for these volunteers, at least, they would in some way be changed forever. I too got a wake-up call in that makeshift MASH unit. It was time to put my angst over Janet's death behind me. It was time to stop going through the motions and get back to work.

Soon after rounds finished, the ambulances and tap-taps began ar-riving with more survivors – an old man with his femur sticking through his skin, a child with two broken arms and so it went. Volunteers from Miami-Dade Fire Rescue brought in a thirteen year old girl who had been pinned in a crevasse inside a crumbled building for four days. They had to dig a tunnel to reach her and then amputate her right forearm on-site in order to free her. It was a day of one miraculous rescue after another. Those miracles came with a price, however, for our census kept growing. New, critically ill patients arrived by the hour, while the few patients stable enough to be discharged, under normal circumstances, had no place to go.

After years of doing primary care in Haiti, it was at first disconcerting to be thrown in the midst of so much trauma. I soon found my niche, however, with plenty of lacerations to stitch, wounds to clean or dress and I.V.'s to start or change. As a competent Creole speaker, I was in constant demand to translate. My first shift, therefore, passed in what seemed an instant. At 8:00 pm, Marie sent me to the airport to await the next plane coming in from Miami

After the intensity of our first few hours in our "MASH unit" it seemed weird to be standing and waiting on the tarmac again. "They also serve who only stand and wait," I told myself and so I stood. The wait seemed extraordinarily long. The plane was supposed to arrive at 8:30. Now it was 10:00. I noticed all the media teams had lights on and cameras aimed at a spot clearly saved for a plane soon to arrive. I drifted towards that spot, eyes trained vainly on the runway, searching for the lights that would signal the arrival of our plane and struck up a conversation with a soldier.

"What's up?" I asked, after introductions.

"We're waiting for some dignitary," the soldier explained. "It happens every night. I hate it. The relief flights get held up for hours while these planes get clearance. Tonight it's some doctor from Boston."

The soldier did not know it but "some doctor from Boston" was actually Dr. Paul Farmer, the doctor and Harvard professor depicted in Tracy Kidder's best-selling book, "Mountains Beyond Mountains." Farmer was now Deputy to the Special Envoy of the United Nations to Haiti. Among the entourage waiting on the tarmac, I saw Loune Viaud, the administrator of Paul's hospital in Haiti, who has long worked with

Project Medishare. Loune is unflappable, thoughtful, always helpful, while at the same time upbeat and optimistic – proof of my theory (to be expounded later) of the need for such altruistic people if our species is to survive.

"Loune," I whispered as I approached her from behind. She turned, we hugged, held hands and gazed into each other's eyes. "Is your family o.k.?" I inquired. "How are things in Cange?"

"My family is fine, thank God, but Cange is another story," she said. "We're already being inundated with patients fleeing Port au Prince. How these patients with broken bones and crushed bodies survive that ride up there – the last hour of road is still unpaved – amazes me, but they do."

"Yes, Marie tells me we've got the same phenomenon in Thomonde and Hinche. I've heard some are traveling as far as Cap Haitian seeking care."

After I told Loune about our field hospital, she introduced me to the reporters accompanying her. "They're from '60 Minutes.'" she explained. "They've come to interview Paul."

"This must be killing him – to be trapped in the States most of the time and forced to deal with the bureaucrats and media at a time like this!" I shouted, over the roar of airplane engines.

Paul had labored in Haiti for more than twenty years, following the injunction of liberation theology to give a "preferential option" to the poor. Lately he had also been working in Rwanda and Peru. The story of his life, "Mountains Beyond Mountains" catapulted him to fame, making him veritable rock star of global health while bringing in millions of dollars to his organization, Partners in Health.

"Come say hi," Loune suggested as the plane finally taxied in. "He'll be thrilled to see you."

When I first met Paul, I think he had his doubts about well-meaning Americans, if not me personally. When we met on my first trip to Thomonde, he wasted no time in admonishing me, "Don't come, make promises and then leave, like so many others, Art, you'll break the people's hearts. You'll smash their hope…"

I promised him then that Project Medishare would stay. Now sixteen years of engagement in Haiti positioned us to help the country deal with this catastrophe.

"No, Loune, there's too much going on and I have to wait for our next group of volunteers to arrive. Just give him my love and let him know Medishare is here, now and for the long haul."

7

Security

Five days after the quake, conditions at the camp approached tolerability. Water and food were flown in daily, along with fresh volunteers, medicines, and supplies for patient care. In fact, we had, if anything, an overabundance of volunteers and supplies. Supplies were packed as high as Alonzo could lift them in an area about ten feet wide and fifty feet long beside the first tent. We had discovered an actual flushing toilet and shower about four hundred yards away, on the edge of the UN compound, which we discretely slipped away to before and after each shift.

The sickest patients had been either triaged out to the Dominican Republic, evacuated to Miami, been operated on, stabilized, or died. We knew our patients by then, as well as their families, who, as is the custom in Haiti, pitched in with feeding, lifting, transporting and assisting with their family members' daily toilet. Children with simple fractures and mild injuries were actually laughing and playing with one another.

For me, the camaraderie I sensed on our first day was further enhanced by the arrival of Project Medishare veterans and other former students and residents. Dan, the very first medical student I took to Haiti fourteen years ago, is now a surgeon. His wife Junia, Haitian-American, who used to be my secretary and was now a physician's assistant, accompanied him. Dan, a Jewish guy from New Jersey, fell in love with Haiti on that first trip and also fell in love with Junia. As her father had died when she was young, I gave her away at their wedding. She calls me "dad," much to the consternation of the other volunteers, who don't know our story. Rudy, the first Haitian-American student I took to Haiti was also among the first volunteers. He had impressed me as a second year student when he correctly diagnosed meningitis in a six month old. I loved working with him during his residency at Jackson Memorial Hospital. We had lost touch after he graduated. The earthquake brought us together.

Then there was Toni, a Haitian-American of the next generation. She was in her last year of our special residency program for social justice and health equality. Her knowledge of Kreyol and her passion to serve her people made her a natural leader in our tent, in spite of her youth. Eddie, another of my former students, now on our faculty as a cardiologist and Director of International Medicine, had returned to being a generalist, changing dressings and I.V.'s like the rest of us.

That night, when they returned from the briefing, Barth and Enrique gathered us around.

"We're going to have to move out of here!" exclaimed Enrique.

"Yeah! They're kicking us out!" added Barth, dejected.

"You're kidding," and "why?" was heard from several quarters.

"They've got rules about security. No Haitians are allowed inside the compound. They see our patients as a breach of security," Enrique continued.

"So this six year old is a security risk?" asked Dan, sarcastically, pointing to a young girl with casts on two broken legs, "and the 'singer'? Yeah, she's a terrorist, alright!"

"We can't fight it." Barth continued. "It's their compound. They say they want us out by 8:00 am on Saturday, but I think that's just their negotiation position. I think they'll let us stay until we find a new home — they just want to motivate us. I'm talking with the government about some land outside the compound. We'll just need to find our own tents."

Alonzo looked disturbed when he heard that our government would not allow critically ill Haitians into the U.S. He was even more distressed to hear that we would have to move. I could tell that he was bonding with the people of Haiti. I suspected he would find unknown spiritual roots in Haiti, just like I had. He was becoming a Vodouisant.

8
From the Arms of Death

Kathie Klarreich was growing restless. She was a free-lance journalist in search of a story in the surreal landscape of a devastated city. She had made the right decision to leave the airport journalism pool, where nothing was really happening. She was witnessing the mushrooming of the Project Medishare field hospital. But so were lots of other reporters. Unlike a lot of these reporters, she spoke Kreyol. She had her own car and driver. Her instincts told her that the real breakthrough story lay "out there," in the rubble, in a place that the visiting journalists unfamiliar with Haiti, would never find or be afraid to go to.

On day five Kathie hatched a plan to follow one of the search and rescue teams that were bringing in survivors to the field hospital regularly. She would offer up her translating skills and knowledge of the local topography in exchange for the opportunity to slip away from the U.N.

compound and see the damage the earthquake had wrought first hand. Her restlessness was fueled by a certain sense of urgency – earthquake survivors were not supposed to survive beyond 72 hours without food and water and there was a danger that any day now, given that fact, search and rescue missions would be cancelled.

The team she would follow had been assigned to canvas the neighborhood of Canapé Vert, on the opposite side of the Capitol from the airport. The journey there afforded her the opportunity to see the destruction on a scale that few other reporters, who tended to go to sites of convenience, had witnessed. She struggled to maintain her journalistic objectivity as her driver passed through neighborhood after neighborhood of the city she had grown to love, now almost totally destroyed. People were gathered in crowds in every open space, while young men and women attempted excavation of pancaked buildings with their bare hands. Down Avenue Haile Selassee, through the slums of Cité Militaire, up the working-class neighborhoods of Delmas. In the Central District with its schools and ministries it was all the same – block after block of rubble. It was no different in the once more upscale environs of Canapé Vert – with the exception of the hospital, and an occasional wood-frame building, there was little recognizable.

The dogs were the first out of the search and rescue trucks, full of canine enthusiasm to start their mission. They were trained to identify both living and dead humans by their scents, a rescue-worker had told Kathie. As she exited her truck, however, she wondered how that could be possible, with the smell of death being so overwhelming. Dogs and workers methodically probed each pile of rubble down one street and up another. As the hours passed, Kathie's suspicion that the time to find survivors might have passed seemed to be confirmed. She drifted away from the search and rescue teams, striking out on her own towards a huge pile of debris up the street. Even after five days, no relief crews had arrived in this neighborhood with food or water. People were combing through the rubble, therefore, scavenging for survival.

Suddenly, one of the scavengers noticed a tiny foot at the bottom of the hole he was excavating. It moved! He began digging furiously. The next thing Kathie saw was the silhouette of a man holding an infant up in the air with one hand. *"Li vivan!"* ("She lives") he shouted, probably assuming the approaching *blan* was a rescue worker. Kathie took the child in her arms, explaining to the onlookers in Kreyol that she'd take the child to a hospital as she ran down the hill to her waiting car and driver. Even a non-medical person could easily tell this poor infant was barely clinging to life. In fact, she panicked for a brief moment that the child might die in her arms.

"Where to?" her driver asked.

"We better go back to the Project Medishare hospital," she said. "At least they have doctors there. It's her only chance."

9

Miwak

"Fifteen minutes, fifteen minutes is all you've got!" the pilot screamed, in a voice loud enough to be heard over the roar of the four turbo props powering the cargo plane to our immediate left. "I want to help, but the Army's running the show here now, and I've only got a half-hour to turn this plane around. You're halfway through that window. Be here in 15 minutes and we'll take her. After the door closes, there's nothing I can do!"

Ninety minutes earlier, someone brought in an infant, six to eight weeks old, to our MINUSTAH triage hospital. I didn't know then where she came from – by the time I finished with the patient I was attending and responded to the commotion, the resuscitation drill was well underway. The two Karens (Karen the pediatrician from Baltimore and Karen the nurse from Miami) worked with marvelous synchrony.

The pediatrician rapidly performed a physical assessment, calling out her findings, while the nurse checked her vital signs, her blood sugar and set up an I.V.

"Depressed skull-fracture... left facial weakness... flail chest..."

"Pulse barely palpable... Apical rate 60... respirations 32... Blood sugar 30..."

I peered around the shoulder of the CNN cameraman, already filming the resuscitation attempt, to witness the object of all this attention. It was an infant – apparently about 2 months old, barely alive, so dehydrated that its skin was as wrinkled as the face of a wizened old farmer. It struggled to cry, too weak to emit a sound and too dry to shed a tear.

"This one's going to be tough to save," I thought to myself, not wanting to distract or discourage the two Karens.

"Her veins are too collapsed for a regular I.V., we'll need an I.O. (intra-osseous line)!" barked Karen the pediatrician.

"Already set up behind you. I brought some with me from Miami."

Karen the pediatrician cleaned the child's thigh with disinfectant then forced a large-bore needle into the bone marrow of the child's femur.

"You've got return!" chimed Karen the nurse, ecstatically.

"Good, let's run it wide open for a bit, and push an amp of D-50 (a concentrated sugar solution)."

"It's running sluggishly. I.V.'s need more height than we can get from this clothesline. Mr. Mourning would you mind holding this bottle as high as you can? Once we get some fluid into her through her bone marrow we'll be able to start a regular I.V."

Alonzo had also come over to see what the fuss was about. His eyes widened as he gazed upon the pathetic sight of a dying infant and widened further in admiration of the resuscitation team's effort. Now he had a role to play. If, as the old saying goes, "success has a thousand fathers," Alonzo Mourning – basketball star now human I.V. pole, could now claim partial paternity.

It would take a few minutes to see how the child responded to the concentrated sugar solution and fluids, so it was a good, non-disruptive time to inquire as to what we knew about this infant.

Me: "Where'd she come from?

Dr. Schneider: "I don't know. She just kind of arrived. Perhaps Search and Rescue. She was so moribund I didn't ask many questions. Evidently, she was found in the arms of her dead mother."

Me: "Great. Just what Haiti needs is another orphan. What's her prognosis? She's looking a little better now. Her facial weakness is improving. Perhaps it's because her blood sugar's rising"

Dr. Schneider: "Yeah, or perhaps because her blood pressure is coming up also. My big concern is she'll tire out. She's got a flail chest and is breathing thirty two times a minute. We've got no oxygen and no Pedi-ventilators. She needs a Pedi-ICU. Without that, she'll poop out and die."

Me: "How much time do we have?"

Dr. Schneider: "A few hours…"

As Karen and I engaged in this conversation the infant in front of us kept getting better. Her heart rate was coming up; her pulse was stronger; a repeat blood sugar had rebounded to 237. The child's biggest problem now was her respiratory distress, which assuredly would exhaust her, and her skull fracture – we didn't know if she was bleeding underneath it. She needed a CAT scan of the brain, a pulse oximeter, some oxygen, and perhaps a respirator – not to mention round-the-clock intensive care and monitoring. We had none of these things. In short, she needed a Pedi ICU. There were none in all of Haiti. The closest was in Miami, seven hundred miles away. Barth and Enrique were away at a Health Cluster meeting leaving me as the most senior physician. What to do?

In that relative calm between the initial resuscitation and the time necessary to await results, everyone who witnessed the child's recovery rallied around to consider our next step. That included the resuscitation team, including Jennifer Ashton (obstetricians are trained in infant resuscitation), who started the peripheral I.V., the camera and reporting crews of CBS and CNN and Alonzo Mourning. What would happen if we just kept her with us? She'd eventually tire and die of respiratory failure. Were there Pedi-ICU's we could send her to? No. Could we evacuate her to the Dominican Republic or Martinique? Not until morning and by then, it would probably be too late. It became increasingly clear that the child's only hope lay in getting her to Miami.

Volunteers started arriving, asking me what they should do. It then dawned on me – if we had new volunteers, then we had to have a plane on the runway. If I hurried, and if all ducks fell in a row, we could send this child to Miami, to our Pedi-ICU at Jackson Memorial Hospital. She'd have a chance there. More than a chance – it was a matter of life or death.

There were two ways to get our airplane- one, passing through two check points, would take me directly to our plane on the tarmac. Project Medishare's driver chose the alternative route, on the public road out the U.N. compound to the airport terminal's main entrance. It would be the faster route, he conjectured, as it would not involve U.N. security clearance. In fact, we made the 1.5 km journey in less than five minutes. The sole entry to the airport, however, was guarded by U.S. soldiers and surrounded by a crowd of Haitians clamoring futilely for access – only U.S. citizens were allowed in. I shouted in Kreyol that I needed to get through to save the life of a Haitian child. Miraculously, the crowd silenced itself and let me pass through. I waved my passport at a soldier to get his attention and explained my need to get to our plane as quickly as possible. Soon, I was sprinting through the abandoned airport and down the tarmac as quickly as my sixty two-year old legs could carry me, followed by my armed escort, in full military regalia.

I flagged down a U.N. driver. She could get me through the checkpoints and save me the few precious minutes I'd need to return to our car. I told her I needed to save the life of a baby.

"What's your name?" I asked.

"Patricia" she answered,

"Get us back here in fourteen minutes and we'll name the baby after you – if she survives!"

"You're on."

The road back to the compound skirted the tarmac, past relief planes from Canada and Israel and around the tents of the Mexican and Colombian relief crews. Patricia radioed ahead to the checkpoints, tooted her horn, and waived away the other trucks along the way. The trip in took seven minutes. She turned the car around while I ran in and gathered the baby and the team.

"Let's go! Let's go! Let's go!" I screamed as I ran in. "We've got a plane, but it will leave in seven minutes."

Stunned by our sudden appearance, Karen, the Pedi-nurse, ran for her passport and gear – she'd be the one to actually accompany the child to Miami – while Karen, the pediatrician, grabbed up the IV bottles and tubing, swaddled the baby in a blanket and ran for the car.

Sitting next to the window on the passenger side, I would carry the I.V. bags for the return trip, while Karen the nurse carried the baby behind me.

"Keep those bags as high in the air as you can" advised the pediatrician. We sped to the airport, Patricia pointing to my arm holding the two I.V. bags to help clear our traffic on the road. In five minutes we lifted the child onto the plane.

"You'll need to fly close to sea level. We don't want her to drop a lung at high altitude!" I explained to the pilot, as the two Karens got the baby settled in on the plane. As the plane taxied down the runway – I used my blackberry to call Carole, our nurse coordinator in Miami. "We're sending a sick child back on the flight leaving now. Skull fractures, flail chest. Five days in rubble. Please have an ambulance at the airport and arrange for admission in the Pedi-ICU."

"No problem!" was Carole's immediate reply.

Carole e-mailed me four hours later. "Things at the airport went flawlessly. She's in the ICU and she looks good! The skull fracture is small and there's little bleeding. The doctors say we got her just in time! The prognosis is good! She should be moved out of ICU in just few a days." I passed this report on to our team. The news was greeted with cheers and tears.

There were lots of reasons I didn't sleep that night. Our teams were packed like sardines on a small platform in front of our patients' cots. Despite our supply of morphine, some of the victims still moaned in pain throughout the night. And they were the lucky ones who got to us for treatment. What about the tens of thousands of injured still scattered about the city? I also, like Enrique, suffered from the adrenaline rush that's slow to subside when you've been dealing with crisis after crisis. I had to make sense out of this baby's story.

Why did this baby survive? Why did she live and all these other kids die? There was a catharsis in her rescue but it wasn't at all clear what it meant. This child's remarkable survival had come about because of a virtually impossible series of events. A child with a strong heart and a will kept herself alive in the rubble for five days without her mother's milk or water. A stranger found her. A journalist looking for a story helped deliver the baby to health care professionals who knew how to stabilize such a survivor. Our team had the two Karens, and CBS reporter/doctor Jennifer Ashton, who had the range of skills needed to revive her. Those health givers had access to high-technology necessary for success. We had a U.N. driver willing to break the rules and take the child to the airport. We had a plane waiting on the runway and a bed waiting at the Pedi-ICU at Jackson Memorial Hospital in Miami. If any one of these particulars had been absent from the equation, the baby would have died. Such a defiance of odds must have meaning.

Scientists and mathematicians have a name for it – an event so improbable that it takes the largest number ever written, a number called a "googleplex," to calculate the odds of it happening. Such an improbable event is called a "googleplex phenomenon." For those who believe that all is explained by the random collision of molecules, googleplex phenomena are the answer to the eternal question, "Why?"

A book might spontaneously leap off the table – a highly improbable but not impossible occurrence that would happen if all the Brownian molecular motions that usually cancel each other out all, by the laws of chance, aligned in the same direction. In the fullness of time, googleplex phenomena will happen. Some will see the story of the rescue of this baby and resuscitation as such an event. With three million people affected and more than a quarter million dead, someone had to beat the odds, and baby Jenny was that person.

Haitians have a different way of explaining highly improbable events. There is no Kreyol word for "disaster." The same word, *"miwak"* (from the French, "miracle") describes an event so extraordinary that it can only be explained as an act of God. In this way of thinking, there is meaning, and ultimately good to be found in the earthquake, its casualties, and its miraculous survivors. That's why Haitians that night were already singing and praying in our field hospital. So what was this baby, anyway – a googleplex phenomenon or a *miwak?* In fact, this child's rescue was beyond miraculous. She was destiny's child. For that matter, my own presence in the field hospital and my role in the child's salvation was also an extraordinary thing – a journey that began more than thirty years before the quake, when I first confronted a mysterious illness in patients who happened to be Haitian, a journey that some would consider absurd. After all, why should a tenured professor with a secure job in Miami care at all about the people in a country many considered cursed? I retraced this tortuous journey in my mind – step by stumbling step. Was my odyssey merely the product of random molecular collisions, or was it also a *miwak?*

Part II
Secrets of the Zombie Curse

10
The Curse Descends

So, how did I get involved in Haiti? In the late 1970s and early 1980s two diseases crept into my professional and personal lives that would change both forever. The first was the newly emerging AIDS virus, a germ that has proven smarter than most of the doctors trying to fight it. The second was one that seemed even more difficult to conquer.

Nothing in my background, education, or training could have prepared me for the misery and mysteries that I experienced in treating the Haitian victims of AIDS starting in 1979. I grew up in a Catholic family of might descent just north of Boston. My father was French Canadian and my mother Italian. For all its veneer of cosmopolitan liberality, Boston is arguably the most provincial city in the United States, particularly in the blue-collar neighborhoods of my youth. At that time Boston was de facto segregated. Black people were hardly ever seen in our neighborhood, even though it was poor. Haiti was unheard of, and Haitian people were completely unknown. In college I was vaguely aware of the rise of "Papa Doc" Duvalier and the Ton Ton Macoutes, but Haiti was a minor issue compared to Vietnam, the Cold War, and civil rights. I did not even know that Haiti was overwhelmingly black, peopled by descendants of the world's only successful slave revolt.

My immigrant Boston blue-collar upbringing was also quite proper. Openly gay people were rarer in our neighborhood than Haitians. But it was the AIDS epidemic, more than anything else that brought homosexuality out of the American closet. Ignorance of the gay experience was a significant contributor to the confusion that physicians--myself included--experienced when AIDS first surfaced in New York City, San Francisco, and Miami in the late 1970s. Even then homosexuality was usually considered a perversion or a psychiatric disease, not only by society at large but also by most of us in the medical profession.

During my internship and residency at the Jackson Memorial from 1973 to 1976 Haitian patients were a rarity. Occasionally, a Haitian merchant seaman would be let off a ship and admitted with malaria or a migrant worker would develop dysentery. That was about it. When poor people in Miami get really sick, they have no alternative but to go "Big Jake," which is supported by Miami Dade County and obligated to treat county residents regardless of their ability to pay. The hospital relied on the University of Miami School of Medicine to provide its workforce. It was a good marriage. The hospital provided an almost-inexhaustible supply of challenging cases, and the medical school provided a small army of faculty members to supervise the residents who cared for the county's poor. All told, over five hundred faculty members and nine hundred residents worked on the campus.

After two years of practice in rural Virginia, I was offered a faculty position at the University of Miami School of Medicine. That's when my Haitian education began. My responsibilities included teaching on the wards and running the medical clinics where Haitian patients were a daily fact. I learned that more than 150,000 Haitians had arrived in Miami during the two years I had been away. Because of their undocumented status and their poverty, most Haitians tended to wait until they were desperately ill before coming to the hospital. It was difficult to get to know them because of their unusual language, a mixture of old French vocabulary with African grammar and syntax.

There was discussion at work as to whether they really sailed from Haiti to Miami in their handcrafted, open sailboats. Some thought they flew to the Bahamas and then were crammed into boats at so much per head and towed across the gulf by organized smugglers. When pressed, however, the people who felt this way could produce no proof other than incredulousness that anyone could survive a journey under such adverse conditions, or the fact that their clothes were always so neat and pressed when they arrived. The Haitians later told me that their tradition was to always bring a carefully wrapped and protected change of clothes to mark their arrival and make a good impression in America. Ironically, those clean, neatly pressed clothes often reflected the colors that characterize one of the island nation's most intriguing contradictions, blue and white, symbolic of Christianity, and red and black, symbolic of voodoo.

At the time, I had a sailboat which I kept moored at a public marina in Crandon Park on Key Biscayne. For a time the Coast Guard kept all confiscated Haitian vessels there, lashed together two or three to a mooring. I would have to row past them in my dingy to get to my boat. They averaged thirty-five feet in length, with brightly painted wooden hulls, fine lines, broad beams, and hand-hewn tree trunks for masts. Landing on our beaches, each boat carried sixty to eight people. Although the boats were handsomely crafted examples of folk art, it seemed incredible that they had survived an ocean crossing. I could not imagine that many people traveling seven hundred miles in such an open vessel. One day I rowed over to one for a closer look. When I peered over the gunwales, I saw the inside of the hull, stained with the grim but unmistakable colors of diarrhea, blood, and vomit. What drives these people to risk such an ordeal? I wondered. And how many people have died completely unknown in the passage?

Looking back, I believe that the faculty of the University of Miami's School of Medicine fulfilled our obligations to our patients in the traditional manner of medical education. We dissected our patients' signs and symptoms and focused on diagnosis and treatment. We were, however, often naive as to whom our patients really were as people. We knew them more as repositories of disease. We were not the only physicians to struggle against a cultural or socioeconomic gap. These gaps are built into our medical system. Few challenge them, and few expect more from their physicians than just to know medicine. In fact, I would learn that the socioeconomic divisions between doctors and their patients enabled the virus that causes AIDS to outsmart us at every turn.

As a group, my Haitian patients struck me as gentle, friendly, and willing to work at practically anything, particularly if it allowed them to "make it" in the United States. There was much discussion about the "Haitian phenomenon" among my colleagues and friends. Most believed that only the brightest and those most driven to succeed were able to gather the resources that allowed them to escape to Miami. Life supported by a menial job in this country was superior to a "middle-class" existence in poverty-stricken Haiti, the poorest country in the hemisphere. However, few of my colleagues knew any Haitians. I did not. My knowledge of them remained superficial, limited to what was necessary to meet their medical needs.

My generation of physicians grew up in an era of antibiotics, believing that all infectious diseases were conquerable. The ability to cure, which we took for granted, was in truth a limited and transient victory for medicine, with a huge downside: It made us lazy. In reality we can prevent illness, we can diagnose, we can ameliorate symptoms, and we can prolong life, perhaps dramatically. To a certain extent we can predict the future, but we can rarely cure. Even when we can cure, many are left behind and that is an injustice.

The second disease I encountered in my medical career was more spiritual than physical. It took my experiences in Haiti to awaken me to the reality of this metaphysical malady, which I call "the zombie curse," as it afflicted my patients, my profession, and myself.

11
Morts et Mysteres

By early 1980 I sensed that something strange, different, and desperate was happening to some of our Haitian patients. Before 1980, spectacular illnesses caught our attention for teaching purposes, like an exploding firework, and faded just as quickly. Gradually, however, several faculty members simultaneously realized that what was happening to some Haitians was different from the rare, sporadic illnesses that had presented themselves to our training program. The patients with these diseases were "classics," behaving in accordance with the classic laws of medicine. But there was nothing classic about what was happening to the Haitians. Some of their illnesses defied all the rules, both in their severity and in the manner of presentation. At first we ascribed the severity of the illnesses to known problems in developing countries-- poverty, malnutrition, and tuberculosis. By early 1980, however, there were just too many facts emerging to let us continue in our complacency.

The illnesses were so bizarre that Lynn, the chair of family medicine, invited a voodoo priest to consult with him. "It can't hurt," he explained, "and some truly believe they have a spell cast on them." Word of this consultation spread rapidly through the medical center. While Lynn already had a reputation as being something of an eccentric, the voodoo priest episode only cemented that impression among most of his peers. To me the patients with these strange illnesses seemed terribly frightened, and medical science had little to offer them to assuage their fears. Lynn may have been on to something after all.

The first person, I met who, in retrospect, had AIDS, acquired immunodeficiency syndrome, came into the general medical clinic on a Wednesday afternoon sometime in the fall of 1979. One of the residents who was scheduled to see patients that afternoon fell ill unexpectedly, and I was helping out by seeing some of his patients. One of them, Jean Baptiste, had just been discharged from the hospital two weeks earlier with the diagnosis of tuberculosis. Since we had effective treatments for tuberculosis, he was supposed to be getting better, but he wasn't. He was emaciated, he could barely walk, and when he did, he fell to one side. His face drooped on the left, and he had signs of spasticity which indicated that something was the matter with his central nervous system.

When I told the senior emergency room resident that I was sending a patient down to be admitted, my presentation was greeted with the kind of skepticism that only a hectic day in our emergency room could generate.

"You've got to give him time to heal, Art. You've got a biopsy-proven diagnosis. He just needs enough time to get better."

When I insisted that he be admitted, the resident finally gave in and said: "O.K. Send him down and we'll take care of him." One week later Jean Baptiste came back to the clinic, having been discharged from the emergency room. By this time he was too weak to walk and had to be assisted by friends. This time I forced his admission on the emergency room with the threat of disciplinary action.

Jean Baptiste was admitted to Lanny's ward team. Lanny, in addition to being my division chief, was also the director of the training program. In those days we used to carpool to work together. While riding into work the following morning I mentioned the case of Jean Baptiste as an example of the tribulations of junior faculty dealing with know-it-all senior residents. Returning home that evening, Lanny informed me that Jean Baptiste was certainly gravely ill and wondered about the possibility of tuberculosis meningitis. Two days later Lanny told me that a CAT scan of Jean Baptiste's brain showed several large lesions. The working diagnosis was tuberculomas of the brain, a rare localized collection of tubercular pus. Over the next two weeks Jean Baptiste continued to deteriorate and finally died despite heroic efforts on the part of Lanny's ward team. Lanny's assessment was that he just had too much disease and had come in too late. This seemed like a reasonable explanation at the time. The story of Jean Baptiste became another vignette for me to pass on to my colleagues as we traded stories of the amazing illnesses that were all too frequently populating our wards.

Over the next several months these horror stories traded among the faculty over coffee or between case presentations in the clinic clearly seemed to involve a disproportionate number of Haitians. Nearly all of them had tuberculosis, not the usual kind involving the lungs but tuberculosis that spread through the lymph nodes, the liver, or throughout the whole body. We all had cases of tuberculosis discovered in the tonsils or under the vocal cords, by liver biopsy, or by spinal tap. We were amazed that a disease we thought we knew so well could behave so virulently. But it still remained a phenomenon, a spectacular disease caused by a particularly virulent strain of tuberculosis, perhaps compounded by malnutrition, and living in close quarters. Many would temporarily get better with treatment. Some developed strange neurological symptoms or superimposed pneumonia. These patients invariably died.

I don't remember who among the faculty first suggested that we group together to study the problem. We all shared a vague sense that something important was going on. Little did we know it would be the greatest medical mystery of our lifetimes. With the exception of Gordon from infectious diseases, we were all from general medicine. Danny and Mark worked closely with me in our particular part of the training program. Art P. was older than the rest of us and had a background in pulmonary medicine, before joining general medicine two years previously. Margaret was junior to Art P., Gordon, and myself. Margaret, who would become a leading AIDS researcher, soon took an informal leadership role in the project. Robby, one of our chief residents, rounded out the group.

Soon we were meeting on a regular basis. Already we had each come to the independent conclusion that disease fostered by poverty and neglect did not completely explain the unusual illnesses we were seeing. These were men and women from various walks of life--housewives, students, and migrant laborers. The only thing they seemed to share was the fact that they had emigrated from Haiti. We all had theories. I was most interested in why tuberculosis was not confined to the lungs, as is usually the case, but rather spread throughout the body. Art P., who knew a lot about tuberculosis, was not impressed with this. He thought disseminated tuberculosis was always more common in younger populations. Danny was interested in how malnutrition might explain what was happening. Mark and Gordon were more interested in the various kinds of unusual infections.

We decided to review all Haitian admissions during the previous year according to a clinical research protocol. In addition to tuberculosis, several unusual infections were documented. Strangely, a single patient frequently had more than one unusual infection. Some patients received an autopsy after they died. We were surprised to find that what we had assumed to be tuberculosis was frequently a parasitic infection of the brain.

New information began falling into place. Fungal infections of the central nervous system, other infections that usually affect only cancer patients receiving chemotherapy, and disseminated viral infections were discovered by our review. My focus on the question of tuberculosis clearly was too narrow. Our patients were behaving as if their immune systems weren't working. Our suspicions grew further when the pathologists began reporting Pneumocystis pneumonia in biopsy and autopsy specimens. Pneumocystis is an amoeba-like organism that only infects patients with weakened immune systems.

By early 1981 our review of the Haitian patients admitted during the previous year showed that the men and women who developed unusual infections were young, had lived in the United States for several months to a few years, were not malnourished before they became ill, and worked in a variety of occupations. They all had blood tests that showed they had previously been exposed to several viruses, including hepatitis, and frequently, but not always, the germ that caused syphilis. In addition to disseminated tuberculosis, a majority had yeast infections in their mouths and swollen lymph nodes in several parts of their bodies. The list of infections we discovered was impressive: viral infections of the esophagus, disseminated herpes virus, disseminated fungal infections, central nervous system fungal and viral infections, central nervous system parasitic infections (toxoplasmosis), and Pneumocystis carinii. Frequently, two or more of these infections were found in the same patient.

It was Margaret who first made the connection between what we were seeing in our Haitian patients and the recently reported occurrence of opportunistic infections in previously healthy homosexual men. Once pointed out, the similarities were indeed striking. But the two groups were not completely alike. First, we had heterosexuals, including women. Second, our patients had much more tuberculosis and toxoplasmosis and much less Pneumocystis pneumonia. We had only one case of Kaposi's sarcoma, a previously rare cancer emerging in the gay population. Still, we knew we were on to something, and began meeting weekly.

Margaret remarked that the problem was being reported more and more in gay men. "It even has a diagnostic category for billing. They're calling it the acquired immunodeficiency syndrome."

The Haitian AIDS mystery began to unfold.

12
Clairvoyante

We decided to follow all new Haitian admissions. Margaret and Art P. drew up a questionnaire, and each of us took turns for a week identifying and reviewing all the Haitians admitted to Jackson Memorial. Any patients who seemed to have the syndrome would be followed by whoever picked them up during his or her week on call. I volunteered my office as a logical place to see patients after they were discharged. It was located behind the medical clinics, and I could arrange for patients to be seen there, regardless of their ability to pay the university's usual private patient fees. While most of our time as medical school faculty was devoted to supervising residents caring for "public" (that is, poor) patients, each faculty member was required to devote a small portion of time to seeing private patients. Dan, Mark, Margaret, and I already saw our private patients there. Fanny and Clara, our secretaries, could facilitate appointments and other logistics. It was clear that these patients could not be well accommodated by the hospital's clinic system, with its long waiting list for appointments and inflexible scheduling.

My week on call finally arrived. The word from those who had already taken call was that I could expect about ten Haitians to be admitted during the week but that only two or three might actually have the syndrome. The most difficult part would be coordinating my schedule with that of the Creole interpreter. Speaking to patients through an interpreter, in their own language, I began to realize how shallowly I knew these people. During rounds I would introduce myself and try to review important historical points in my best college French. The patients would stare at me blankly or answer in English "Yes, yes" and I knew not a single word I had spoken was comprehended. Now I was able to examine their lives in exact and intimate detail. Through their language I discovered their intelligence, emotions, sophistication, and sense of humor. My interest in the research took a back seat to my growing fascination with the patients themselves.

I loved them from the beginning. I loved them because they were underdogs. I loved them for their improbable names: Theophile ("love of God," in Greek), Clairvoyante ("fortune teller"), Marc Aurele (the Roman emperor/stoic philosopher), and Mercidieu ("thanks be to God"). I could trace part of their culture to France, for many of their names—Voltaire and Rousseau, for example-had a hint of the Enlightenment. The language shared with its parent French a rhythm and softness and seemed to have an intrinsic rule that it be spoken while smiling, no matter how much the speaker was suffering. At the same time, I sensed in their speech an Africa of long ago. It sounded like French but was incomprehensible as such and was peppered with repetitive sounds, almost as if it were intended to be danced to, with drumbeats as accents. Their families, particularly, their children, were dressed in a way that surpassed style and approached artistry, even though they were poor. These features of custom and language made them exotic, which enhanced my attraction to them. Poor, peaceful, humble, and hungering after justice, they seemed to be the beatitudes personified.

The house staff was not quite as sanguine in their opinions. They gave whatever was necessary in terms of hours, dedication, and compassion to these patients with overwhelming illnesses. But already Haitian admissions were getting a reputation as "bad hits," and a sort of gallows humor was beginning to emerge. During rounds one day, in response to an uncommonly prejudicial remark by a medical student, I remarked, that I had rarely seen a Haitian admitted with any of the diseases we usually associate with alcohol or drug abuse. One of my interns snorted, "That's because they don't live long enough."

I interviewed a 42-year-old woman whom I will call Josie. It was hard to believe she might have the syndrome, despite her disseminated tuberculosis and telltale oral yeast infection. She looked younger than her age and was slightly overweight. Two years before, she had left her six children in Haiti and come to this country to do domestic work, sending her meager earnings back to her family. She smiled incredulously when I asked through the interpreter if she had ever had a bisexual lover or sex with a woman. Questions about oral sex and anal sex were met with the same look of surprise. Yet Josie was not offended by the questions and answered in a matter-of-fact manner. She had several boyfriends in Haiti before the birth of her first child, but was then monogamous until her husband died and she came to this country. There had been no unusual sexual practices, she said, just ordinary relations between wife and husband.

The only other patient I picked up that first week was named Claude. He was in his mid20s and had come here as a student. Again, I saw the same incredulous smile and disclaimers in response to my questions about homosexuality and sexual practices. He looked much sicker than Marie; he was wasted and suffering from high fever. Still, he was polite and agreeable and seemed glad that someone was taking an interest in his illness.

Blood was drawn, and my forms were completed and passed on to Margaret, who coordinated things, along with my assessment of "one probable, one definite." Claude continued to decline in the hospital and died of toxoplasmosis a few days later. Marie was discharged in reasonably good condition: however, she did not return for her follow-up appointment. Two months later she arrived in the emergency room with overwhelming pneumonia and died within 24 hours. Margaret informed me that my "probable" had become a "definite."

Haitian patients with the syndrome continued to be admitted to my ward team. Previlus presented with fever, diarrhea, and disseminated tuberculosis. He was a slight man, smaller than average but muscular. His hairline had receded, and he kept his hair trimmed close to his scalp. He had somehow found his way to us from Palm Beach County, where he lived and worked as a migrant laborer. He spoke articulate English and French, in addition to Creole. He was the first to complain to me of itchy bumps on his skin. We asked dermatology to see him. The consultant's diagnosis was fleabites, but when informed of this opinion, Previlus protested adamantly.

"I don't have fleas, Docteur."

"I understand, Previlus, but that's what the skin specialists think."

"I am not a dog, Docteur."

"Perhaps they're some other kind of insect bite. You do work in the fields. Perhaps red ants."

"I have never had these before, Docteur. There are no insects on me. I have no fleas."

I let the issue go, not knowing he was right.

The cause of his diarrhea was discovered through the persistence of a fourth-year student rotating through the team, who would not accept my explanation of this problem by conventional causes. He discovered an unusual parasite in Previlus's intestines that was not supposed to cause disease in humans. Previlus was the first patient with AIDS in whom this infection was discovered. Unfortunately, none of our treatments brought him anything more than temporary relief. Although we could not relieve his itching or cure his diarrhea, Previlus did improve enough with treatment of his tuberculosis to allow him to leave the hospital. In fact, diagnosing tuberculosis in its myriad new forms and effectively treating it (it took three medicines for at least nine months) was one of our first real successes.

The old vernacular name for tuberculosis was "consumption," which graphically described how Previlus and the others with tuberculosis looked when they first presented–gaunt and wasted, as if being slowly consumed by a fire burning inside them. Fortunately, after a few days of treatment, Previlus's temperature came down and his appetite improved dramatically. After his discharge, I volunteered to follow him in my office, where he joined Theophile and Marc, two other survivors.

Gordon picked up Theophile when he was admitted with a type of fungal meningitis. When he came to the office he always looked remarkably well, wearing a brightly colored shirt and a broadbrimmed straw hat. He was tall and thin but not wasted and had an infectious grin. He complained of headaches after his meningitis, and Gordon treated him with codeine. Whenever he ran out of medicine he would show up unexpectedly at our office. Since I was there more often than Gordon, I would frequently renew his prescriptions.

Marc was one of the first in whom we diagnosed toxoplasmosis of the brain before he died. Initially he responded dramatically to treatment, but the nursing home he was discharged to inadvertently discontinued it. When he returned to us he was paralyzed on his right side and could not speak. Although restarting antibiotics forestalled his death, the drugs did not restore his strength or his speech. He returned to our office in a wheelchair each week to see Margaret. He smiled on one side of his face and drooled on the other in response to greetings from Fanny and Clara. They mercifully ignored his disability and carried on one-way conversations with him: "Oh, Marc, you're here. The doctor will be right with you. You look like you're doing better."

Despite our patients' marginal health, I was optimistic. It was exciting. The veil of ignorance had been partially lifted. Patients who would have previously died were surviving and leaving the hospital. Many did reasonably well between relapses, despite their blood tests, which showed that they were still immune deficient. We had effective treatments for many but not all of the infections and hoped that if we could buy enough time either we would find a cure or the patients would recover spontaneously.

We also knew something that hardly anyone else knew: This terrible disease did not affect homosexual men exclusively. The speculations in the letters section of the New England Journal of Medicine—that AIDS was related to the recreational drug of amyl nitrate or the immunosuppressive properties of sperm in the bloodstream-were fanciful and wrong. But what was the connection between these Haitians and gay men with the same illness? Was this something new, or had it been there all along but in our ignorance we had missed? We speculated among ourselves. New virus? Mutant virus? Combination of viruses in sequence? Genetic predisposition? Old virus behaving in a new manner? Perhaps it was exposure to malaria or some other parasitic organism endemic to Haiti? Each of these theories was considered, but there were no hard facts to support any of them.

Mary Jo in obstetrics delivered the baby of a pregnant mother dying of tuberculosis. Gwen and Wade in pediatrics followed this child and soon others, some born of seemingly healthy mothers. All eventually succumbed to bizarre infections. So now we had men, women, and children, in growing numbers. Their only link? They were all Haitians.

13
Regis

Dan and I alternated monthly as attending physicians on the in-patient service at Jackson Memorial Hospital. I was about to take over responsibility for the service, and Dan was briefing me on the patients. We had been working together for three years and frequently commiserated about the plight of our patients.

"The sickest is definitely this fellow Regis. Have you heard of him? He was admitted with pneumocystis carinii pneumonia. His blood count started to fall on Bactrim. We stopped it, and we're waiting for pentamidine to arrive from the CDC Centers for Disease Control and Prevention. He's dying fast. You may be forced to restart the Bactrim. It's remarkable. He was a dentist in Haiti."

When I met Regis on rounds the following day he was near death. He had pneumonia throughout his lungs. He was breathing heavily at three times the normal rate and was too weak to talk. His mouth was dry, despite the oxygen mist streaming from a mask over his face, and his eyes were rolled back in his head. When he was admitted his temperature was 105° F. It decreased to 102° while on Bactrim but climbed again when his antibiotic was changed. Because of the glut of terribly sick patients the syndrome was already causing, there were no beds available in the intensive care unit. My resident and I decided we would give the pentamidine one day to work, watch Regis closely, and intubate and artificially ventilate him if necessary. We would not let the absence of an intensive care bed keep us from doing everything we could. After questioning the medical students and answering their questions, my team moved on to the next patient. As sick as he was, Regis was only one of about twenty-five patients under my care.

The next morning Regis was even worse. The intern on call had been up all night with him, restarting intravenous lines, drawing cultures, and frequently checking his arterial blood gases. His chest xray showed more consolidation of the pneumonia, and his blood gases were deteriorating. We decided to give up on the pentamidine and restart the drug he had been on three days before. Bactrim could kill the organism causing Regis's pneumonia more effectively, but it had stopped his bone marrow from making red cells. Now this seemed the lesser of two evils. We could always transfuse him, and we hoped a special vitamin – folic acid would reverse the drug's effect on the bone marrow.

The intern on call was again up all night ministering to Regis. By the following morning he showed signs of improvement. He was breathing more easily and his chest sounded clearer. His temperature had dropped to 101. He had the strength to talk again.

"Who are you?" he asked me as I leaned over to listen to his chest.

"I'm Doctor Fournier. I'm in charge of the team you were admitted to."

"Oh, the name on the bracelet?" he smiled as he pointed to the identification band on his wrist that contained his name, his hospital number, and my name. In a teaching hospital hardly anyone notices the name of the attending physician on the I.D. bracelet.

Even so, after having so recently climbed out of the grave, he was handsome and noble looking. His skin was truly black, unblemished, and shining with the moisture of perspiration and the oxygen mist. His eyes were animated and accentuated by angular cheeks and a broad, sharply crested nose. His teeth were impossibly white and perfectly shaped and spaced. His English was perfect, without a hint of an accent.

There was no doubt he had AIDS. In addition to pneumonia, he had patches of fungus inside his cheeks and on his palate. The number of lymphocytes in his blood counts was depressed, a sure sign, and his "helper" to "suppressor" T cell ratio was inverted. T cells are the part of the immune system that fights off unusual infections. We now know that the AIDS virus specifically attacks the "helper" or "T4" lymphocytes slowly, over time depleting their numbers. When they reach critically low levels, patients become sick with unusual infections. But Regis had no signs of tuberculosis and a test for syphilis was negative. The residents were justifiably proud of pulling him through, especially since they had done it without the benefit of an intensive care bed. Paul, his intern, could not wait for my arrival at rounds the next day.

"Boy, you're not going to believe how much better Regis is today. The man's incredibly smart. He was asking all about his illness, and I told him about the pneumonia, and the Bactrim and the pentamidine and how his immune system is all screwed up. He understands it all. His blood gas is almost normal, and his chest xray's even starting to look better."

"Good morning, Dr. Fournier. How are my T cells doing this morning?" Regis asked when we arrived in his room. He was up in a chair, had washed, and was able to breathe comfortably without the oxygen. I paused for a moment to let the resident bask in their accomplishment.

"Well enough. You have improved greatly."

"Then you think I will recover?"

"You're recovering already."

"But will my T cells recover?"

I would have taken this last question as a joke except that he asked it with complete sincerity. I had never been asked a question of such immunological detail by one of my patients. Clearly, he was seeking reassurance for questions deeper than T cell function. I felt constrained by the format of attending rounds and answered with a trite, "Only time will tell."

I shared the resident's exhilaration in pulling Regis through. Regis had been all but dead three days before. Had he presented as little as six months earlier he surely would have died despite of our efforts, as we wouldn't have had a clue as to the true cause of his pneumonia or the best treatment. His strength increased daily. Soon we incorporated Regis into our rounds, asking him to translate for all our Creolespeaking patients, rather than waiting for the interpreter. He was excellent at this, and reported not only what the patient said but also an assessment of the patient's level of understanding and unspoken concerns. He added a touch of drama and eloquence as he told each patient's story. The patients were puzzled at first as he emerged from the group of physicians and students wearing a hospital gown and pajamas and still attached to an IV pole. But he stated plainly what he was doing and then put them at ease with a smile and a handshake. We all remarked what a luxury it was to have our own interpreter and one of such quality.

Regis seemed different from many of the other Haitian patients. For one thing, no family members ever visited him. He was always reading or writing. His bedside table had only a King James Version of the Bible to adorn it, rather than the usual pictures of saints that graced the tables and walls of other Haitian patients. "Mysterious," I thought.

One day toward the end of his hospital stay I was making rounds alone, dictating my daily notes into a handheld dictaphone. When I got to Regis's room I decided to stop in, since I had missed the opportunity to see him during particularly hectic morning rounds with the team. I knocked and entered. He was reading his Bible.

"Hello, Regis. I didn't get to see you during rounds this morning. Continuing to make progress?"

"Yes, doctor. I think my lymphocytes are holding their own now. Thank you. Won't you visit for a while?" He closed his Bible and placed it on a photo album on top of his bed stand. I accepted his invitation and asked how he had come to this country. He told me he had grown up in the Haitian countryside but had always been a good student at the Protestant missionary school in his village. After high school he took a correspondence course in dentistry, there being no dental school in his part of Haiti, and the mission sponsored him in setting up and running a dental clinic. He did this for five years and even wrote a book for the public on dental hygiene. As he told me this, he pulled the book from his drawer and displayed it with a smile. Now he had come to this country to formalize his education. He both studied and taught English as a second language at a local college. He was thirty-three years old.

The book was in English and was obviously written at a time when Regis's English had not reached its present state of perfection, for it was grammatically but not idiomatically correct. His picture was on the frontispiece, handsome in a three-piece suit. The content concerned fundamentals of caring for teeth the importance of brushing and cleaning and what happens during a visit to the dentist. The mission had published it. He was quite proud of it.

The photo album was of greater interest to me. There were many pictures of Regis surrounded by white people somewhere in the United States. These were his visits to the mission's stateside base. Interspersed with these were photos of him in an obviously tropical setting, usually surrounded by groups of children or adults. But one picture arrested me--Regis in a small, bare room with one chair and an older woman seated in a handmade chair. Regis had one bare hand in her mouth and with the other was extracting a tooth with a pair of pliers. The woman's face was contorted, and her legs were crossed in pain. Remembering cases of dentists with hepatitis, I could not escape the revelation: This was how he had contracted the disease.

I told him how fascinated I was by the pictures of his life in Haiti. He seemed pleased and told me I should visit Haiti someday. He asked me what would become of him. It was clear that the knowledge he had absorbed from Paul's lessons in immunology was more than superficial. But he was calm and not frightened. He said he had to get better so he could finish his education and return to his work in Haiti. I told him that his problem was serious but not hopeless. Several patients had died, but more and more were surviving, and this illness was still too new to predict the future. I offered to follow him in my office and promised that, if the situation did become hopeless, I would tell him.

14
Blood Brothers

It was the early 1980s and the media had discovered the "gay plague." The newspapers carried sensational stories about the unexplained epidemic in the morning. In the evenings, the TV news would have had another. Who could blame them? It was a huge story. The disease was new, contagious, and connected to sex.

Our group studying the Haitian victims of the disease had an important contribution to make to this growing public discussion of AIDS. Having gathered convincing evidence that it was not confined to gay men, we notified the Center for Disease Control of our findings. CDC sent a task force to meet us, saw some of our patients, reviewed our data, and helped us with special immunological testing. We heard from the agency that some patients from the Haitian community in New York City had come down with same illness. We were preparing our data for publication.

For most of us in the original study group, AIDS among Haitians remained a part-time endeavor. Margaret, however, was devoting more and more of her energy to the problem. She followed the largest number of patients and came to the office to see them practically every day of the workweek, instead of the one-half day a week usually devoted to the faculty private practice. She and Art P. were planning a trip to Haiti to look for evidence of the syndrome there. She talked about the subject with urgency and an excitement the rest of us did not share.

Regis was doing the best of the patients I followed. He felt well, his appetite was good, and he was gaining back the weight he had lost during his bout with pneumonia. He would come to the office in a suit and tie, looking like an ambassador. He made light, pleasant conversation with the office staff. For a while he was doing so well that I thought he might be the first spontaneous recovery. But his lymphocyte count remained low, and tests showed that he was still immunodeficient despite his outwardly robust appearance. One bothersome problem was the development on both ankles of the same type of itchy bumps that plagued Previlus. I did not even attempt to offer the dermatologist's explanation of "insect bites" to Regis. Fortunately, since he was so concerned about his appearance, the bumps were hidden beneath his trousers.

Margaret asked me if I knew anyone who had B+ blood type. I answered that I was B+, knowing that in answering I was also volunteering for something. I wondered if she had somehow checked in advance. She wanted to mix the lymphocytes and sera from our Haitian patients with "normals" and inject them into marmosets. Regis was B+, and that being a relatively rare blood type, she had yet to find a "control." "It's only 50 cc's," she demurred. So I drew the blood sample from Regis, and Margaret drew a sample from me. "I guess this makes us 'Sang-frè-yò-blood brothers," said Regis, smiling.

All of these patients required lots of attention and we saw them frequently. The nature of our office waiting room was changing. With the exception of Regis, there was no mistaking that these patients were poorer and sicker than the private patients who shared the waiting area with them. The private patients would consciously or unconsciously sit as far from the Haitians as they could. I'm sure many wondered what they were doing there. If two or more Haitians were waiting, they and their families would chatter in Creole, while the private patients waited silently, with their noses buried in The New Yorker or Sports Illustrated. Sometimes, if a particularly sick Haitian was waiting, a private patient would stare as if seeing an apparition. Still, no overt objections were raised, for the reason the Haitians were there remained a secret.

Now, two or three new cases a week were being admitted to the hospital. Only half survived to be discharged. One corridor of one floor was exclusively occupied by Haitian patients with AIDS. Because they were poor, without resources, frequently living here illegally and unaware that this disease was among them, many arrived at the hospital moribund. The residents continued to work heroically to keep them alive, but the high mortality was eroding morale.

The word was filtering through the hospital that our Haitian patients were suffering from the same disease that the media was calling the "gay plague." The beginnings of the backlash were appearing-transportation workers refusing to escort patients for x-rays; nurses worry about our patients in semiprivate rooms sharing bathrooms with other patients; interns skipping rectal examinations; surgical residents dragging their feet on performing biopsies and necessary operations.

Back at the office, Margaret had started seeing gay men with the syndrome. Although she made no announcement, there was no mistaking the fact by those of us who shared the office. Some were stereotypically openly gay. They dressed effeminately and talked with our secretaries as if they were sisters. Others were recognized only because they came back time and again with the same men. Although some were resigned, and all held up under the strain with remarkable dignity and fortitude, most were anxious. Their anxiety was not helped by Margaret's schedule, which frequently had her in two places at once. There were frequent outbursts of anger as they waited. Some with Kaposi's sarcoma had large, red lesions on their arms and faces that announced to the whole world that they were gay and had AIDS, like a modern-day scarlet letter. Some came with their parents. Others came with their lovers. Occasionally couples would know each other and make pleasant conversation about mutual acquaintances or interests. Usually, however, the mood was somber, especially if there were a particularly sick or wasted patient in the group.

I had many discussions about this new development riding to and from work with Amal. She is an Egyptian Christian physician who lived with an American family in my neighborhood and worked in our office doing research with Mark on hypertension. She was fascinated with everything American, an incurable optimist, and a compulsive storyteller. We were in the habit of having wide-ranging discussions about politics, religion, culture, and morals to pass the time as we commuted. She claimed an intense interest in the mysteries of life, which she attributed to her ancient ancestors, the children of Pharaoh. She looked like Nefertiti, with large eyes and straight black hair. She often told me it was the Christian Egyptians who were the true descendants of Pharaoh, not the Muslims, who sprang from Arab invaders. She held profoundly fundamentalist religious views, steeled by belonging to a religious minority in her own country. She did not believe in evolution, she interpreted the Bible literally, and she held a Calvinist view of fate. Nothing happened unless God willed it.

She had several vignettes she would recount during our rides to work to illustrate God's active intervention in her life. I was such an intervention. Only a beneficent Deity would have arranged for her to live in the same neighborhood as me and to have me pass directly by her home on my way to and from work. In exchange for this gift she felt compelled to convert me from skepticism. Fortunately for me, I had had the opportunity to practice all the religious arguments as I passed through

Catholic high school and college. I therefore took these attempts at conversion as scholastic amusement, while she took them with sincerity and earnestness. On the assumption that the best defense is a good offense, I told her my theory of the homophilic origins of early Christian theology. This theory had been finely honed many years before during free periods in my college canteen. Of course, with all that talk of brotherly love and traveling around with a bunch of guys and never getting married, saying Jesus was gay was an easy next step. But three early followers deserved critical review. Was Judas' behavior that of a lover scorned? Da Vinci thought as much in "The Last Supper." And wasn't St. John the disciple that Jesus loved? Finally, there was Saint Paul. He was a grecophile and a misogynist. By interpreting the experience of Christ in the light of Greek thought, he linked the God of Love forever to Plato, who clearly felt homosexual love was love in its purest form. Such talk both scandalized and titillated Amal. She was intrigued that an American would even think about such matters. My conversion from skepticism became one of her priorities.

She was fascinated by the closeness of some of the gay couples. "They always come in pairs," she remarked to Fanny.

"Just like Noah's ark," I commented, overhearing her whispers. She claimed there was no homosexuality in her country. "Not even among the Muslims?" I countered. She wavered at this and almost took the bait, since she despised the Muslims, but would not concede the possibility of homosexuality among her countrymen. To Amal, AIDS was a punishment visited on the gays for their sins. Better they should suffer here on earth than suffer the pains of eternal damnation. The Haitians were more problematic, but she was unshakable in her belief that their suffering somehow manifested God's glory.

I was not so sure.

15
The Zombie Curse

Dan and I, who were responsible for our residents' education in clinic matters, asked Ginette, a young Haitian-American psychiatry resident, if she would talk to the residents about Haitian culture. We hoped these talks might break down some of the barriers that had surfaced between our residents and their patients. Ginette served as our liaison with the Department of Psychiatry. She usually taught the residents generic issues that general medical doctors need to know about psychiatry—recognizing depression, treating anxiety. The idea of using someone from one culture to teach doctors from another culture was novel. Poised and confident, she set up a television and videocassette recorder and engaged the residents with her eyes.

"Today I'm going to share with you the secret of the zombie curse." Usually it was difficult to get the medical residents involved in behavioral science seminars, but Ginette captured her audience with her first sentence.

"There are zombies in Haiti, and it's related to voodoo," she said. "Who knows what voodoo is?"

"That's the religion in Haiti where they stick pins in dolls," volunteered one resident. "People are so afraid of it, that it controls their minds," another resident answered.

"You've been watching too many movies," said Ginette. "Voodoo is the Creole pronunciation for the French Vieux Dieux the old gods, the spirits of the forest, in Creole the *Lwa's*, who can be called out from their homes in the mapou and mahogany trees. The gods the slaves brought from Africa. The French tried to impose Catholicism and to a certain extent succeeded. But the old gods, the Lwa's, continued almost like the Catholic saints there for personal intervention. In fact, in Haiti many of the saints have two personas their Catholic image and their Voodoo role. The power of the *doktè fè* you might call him a witch doctor, but the name really means 'leaf doctor' comes not from superstition but from a refined knowledge of the pharmacological effects of local plants and animals."

"Just as the Eskimos have many words for snow, the Haitians have several names for practitioners of their secret rites. In addition to *docté fè*, there's *hougan*, which means spell giver; *book*, a male priest; and mambo, priestess. And there are several kinds of spells too, good spells and bad ones, ranging from a *mojo* – a love potion-through curses meant to wreak revenge. The worst, though, is the zombie curse. Ginnette showed a documentary tape from the BBC of people who were declared dead, buried, and then turned up alive. In one case, a man returned to his sister's house fourteen years after he was buried."

The residents were fascinated, and she went on.

"The key to the zombie curse is tetratotoxin, found in the skin of puffer fish, abundant in the waters surrounding Haiti. It induces a state indistinguishable from death. The *doktè fè* returns after the funeral, exhumes the body, and administers an antidote that keeps the zombie in a drugged state. Zombie is Creole for 'like a shadow.' Literally, when you're a zombie, you're only a shadow of your former self."

"The subject of the curse is condemned to a life of slavery, the worst fate possible for the descendants of former slaves. The curse is therefore only applied by a secret village council to individuals believed to have violated the rules of society and who need to be cast out. It was a way of keeping the old religion and indeed the old African society alive, and it served as a potent weapon against their French masters. Think of the symbolism. The *doktè fè* has actual power over life and death. You die, and he raises you up, not just your soul but your body as well. That's tough for other religions to match."

"Great lecture," I thought. "One of the best I've ever heard."

Unfortunately, the audience consisted of only Dan, Amal, six residents, and myself. The residents were enthusiastic and congratulated Ginette for an excellent talk.

"Now that you know about the zombie curse, don't keep it a secret," she advised. "Tell your fellow residents."

On the ride home I asked Amal what she thought of voodoo and the zombie curse. "Only God can give us everlasting life," she responded. "It's magic, black magic, a trick. A clever trick, but a trick all the same."

"I think you missed the point," I said, looking at her and negotiating traffic at the same time. "It's not a question of whether it's magic or real, although that guy who walked into his sister's home 14 years after being declared dead sure seemed real to me. It's a question of whether voodoo is a real religion or not, on the same par with Catholicism, Buddhism, Islam, and all the others. I think Jeannette made a compelling case that it is—a coherent set of beliefs and practices to make sense out of the unknown and perhaps exercise some degree of control over it. The thing about the zombie curse that's so interesting to me is not the spell itself, but the fact that it has the full weight of a law. It's cast as a formal judgment of innocence or guilt."

Amal fell silent for the remainder of the ride home. I think our theological discussions were starting to frighten her.

By the time our paper had been accepted for publication, someone at the Centers for Disease Control had already informed news reporters Haitians were at risk for AIDS. The Miami Herald had a front-page article entitled "Haitians Dying of 'Gay Plague.'

Other stories suggested that AIDS, in fact, originated in Haiti and perhaps was related to secret voodoo ceremonies involving the drinking of blood. These stories, usually accompanied by a picture of a voodoo priest or priestess slaughtering a chicken or goat, I found particularly offensive. The implication was that you could get AIDS from drinking animal blood or that there were secret voodoo ceremonies involving cannibalism, vampirism, or human sacrifice. Even having just begun the process of getting to know a few Haitians as real people rather than media caricatures, these stories infuriated me. I could only imagine how the Haitians felt.

Margaret appeared on television several times attempting to explain what we had discovered, but the media always seemed to edit her meaning. It hurt to see how our work was being distorted and misrepresented in the press. Our discovery of twenty-two patients with AIDS was portrayed as a rising epidemic threatening to engulf the 150,000 Haitian immigrants residing in South Florida. The possibility of heterosexual transmission implied by our data fueled the flames of sensationalism.

Spokesmen, including physicians, in the Haitian community were particularly upset with us. To a certain extent they were justified. Life for Haitian immigrants in Miami was difficult enough without having the entire community accused of introducing a modern-day plague. Haitians were both fired and not hired because the research performed by us played to the inherent bigotry of some employers. The Haitian community responded to this threat to its existence in our country by accusing us of being bad scientists. We hadn't been able to talk to the patients in their native language; we didn't understand the Haitian cultural taboos against homosexuality and therefore the reluctance of our patients to admit to such practices. We had failed to involve the Haitian community in our study. Most of this anger was directed at our most visible representative: Margaret.

Our Haitian critics charged that labeling Haitians as being a risk group for AIDS was just a new sort of racism. Each of these charges, but particularly the last one, hurt us deeply. We had started our project with no preconceived ideas, only the problem of sick patients who happened to be Haitians who were dying on our wards. We never claimed that patients got AIDS because they were Haitian, only that the disease was present in a group whose only apparent link was a common ethnic background, similar to sickle cell anemia among American blacks or ulcerative colitis among Jews. These were medical facts, not political statements: clues to the riddle, not bullets for a gun.

These charges raised the first seeds of doubt about what we were doing. In retrospect we had been naive in our interviewing techniques and our assumption that patients, speaking through interpreter, would reveal intimate details to physicians they had never before met. We probably did not identify some who were gay, or who had sold themselves in prostitution, or who had visited prostitutes but were ashamed to admit it. But for the most part, those men that we followed, overtime who told us they were not homosexual seemed quite credible. And what of the women? How did they get the disease if homosexuality was the only risk factor? In attempting to protect the Haitian community from bigotry, our critics were forced to question not only us but also the truthfulness of each of our patients. It seemed to be a no-win situation.

Then in 1983 and 1984 the whole debate was resolved, at least scientifically. Dr. Luc Montagner in France and Dr. Robert Gallo in the United States respectively, discovered that AIDS was caused by a virus. That discovery made the whole concept of risk factors irrelevant. AIDS was an infectious disease, nothing more. But it was too late. But in the public mind, the labeling, stereotyping, and blaming had already taken hold.

The politicization of AIDS in the press had adverse effects on day-to-day life on the hospital wards. Panic was spreading among the hospital personnel. It seemed like everyone was worried about being infected. Not all but some nurses refused to bathe patients with AIDS, transportation workers refused to move patients with AIDS, and in some cases resident avoided caring for AIDS patients. I would be embarrassed to enter elevators and find patients who obviously had AIDS going to the x-ray department or some other part of the hospital being transported by people wearing surgical gowns, masks, caps, gloves, and booties. In defiance, I made an effort to talk to these patients if I knew them, wish them well, and touch them as we parted company. Walking down the corridors I would overhear nurses' assistants saying to each other things like, "I don't care if they fire me. There is no way I'm emptying so and so's bed pan." I made a point to go up to these groups and tell them not to believe what they were reading in the newspapers. I had touched these patients in the course of examining them as much as anyone, going back to before we even knew the disease existed, and I was still alive and well. Usually my pleas for rationality were met with quiet disbelief.

Pressure was increasing from two directions to try to get me to move Margaret's practice. From the clinic administration I would hear about alleged complaints from the private patients about sharing the waiting room, examining rooms, and bathroom with AIDS patients. Are the examining rooms wiped down with alcohol each time after they're used? Are the toilet seats disinfected? And thank God we have disposable speculums! These objections were easy to deal with. I told the administrators that there was no evidence a person could get AIDS from just sitting where someone with the disease had sat. Margaret was taking care of a problem no one else was willing to face and that was not going to go away. Yes, I agreed, thank God for plastic speculums. (It's hard to believe now, but disposable speculums were still an innovation at Jackson Memorial Hospital in the early 1980s.)

It was more difficult for me to deal with complaints from fellow faculty. They had known of my study from the beginning. They were friends. They were working for the same goals that I was. They cared about our patients. They told me that this was no way to run a private practice. The AIDS patients were never going to be a central part of our job, which focused on teaching general internal medicine. Private practice development was more important. If I wanted the private practice to succeed, the AIDS patients would have to go. One faculty members, who are is usually calm and unflappable, were as particularly upset.

"This office has become Miami's answer to the Turkish baths. Fanny found two gays fondling each other behind the door to her office. How would you feel if you were a private patient sitting in our waiting room and were surrounded by all these homosexuals? And Theophile, he's walking around begging for cab fare home. You have to talk with Margaret."

I told him I would talk to Margaret, but I stalled. Meanwhile, Margaret's composure was beginning to unravel. Although she wouldn't admit it, she clearly had more work than one person could manage. Patients sometimes arrived without appointments, having heard about her through the grapevine. They waited all afternoon just to have the opportunity to talk with her and try to make an appointment. Others with appointments waited all afternoon only to be turned away without seeing her, as she was tied up in the hospital ministering "last rights" to one of her dying charges. The house staff's gallows humor said if you're a patient you know you are in trouble when they call in Margaret as a consultant. Some very cruel colleagues referred to her as the "fag queen."

These sorts of comments, coupled with the criticisms directed at her from the Haitian community, needed only the extra burden of the death of one of her patients to bring her to the verge of tears. On occasion she would blow up at the secretarial staff and then, regaining her composure, apologize. Gwen in pediatrics and Mary Jo in obstetrics were under similar strains—solitary figures fighting a lonely battle against a disease few of their peers wished to face.

16
Revelations

For several weeks in 1984 my mood was clouded by a story I saw on the evening news. The bodies of thirty-two Haitians had washed up on a beach just north of Miami. Their homemade sailboat had broken up at night during a storm only two hundred yards from shore. The images on the screen were both horrible and fascinating. The sailboat was still recognizable, half buried in the sand, with waves breaking over it. With honesty rarely shown by television news, the dead Haitian men and women were shown strewn along the beach almost as if enjoying a holiday. Most were nude and in death beautiful. Their bodies were young and muscular, and their skin was textured by sand and beads of water sparkling under a brilliant sun. They must have died shortly before the cameras arrived, for rigor mortis had not yet set in, and they had not yet become bloated. Each wave would wash over them and then ebb, moving them just enough to make them appear to be still alive. Most were face down, looking perfectly at peace. The next day the television station that carried the story apologized for the graphic footage the night before; they claimed it was a late-breaking story.

A few who survived the ordeal had been taken to the Krome Avenue camp. They told how they had signed up with smugglers for $200 per person and how forty people had crowded into the small open boat and set sail up the Windward Passage to Florida, two hundred yards from shore, just before dawn, a squall capsized the boat. Most were just too weak from the journey to make it the remaining distance. The survivors were not even allowed to attend their shipmates' funerals.

Amal and I discussed the tragedy during our ride home.

"I'm angry with my government for forcing disasters like this to happen and ashamed to be an American," I told her. "Everyone gives lip service to love and freedom and uses them to sell everything from hamburgers to insurance. But when you cut away all the crap, nobody really cares about these people. How many others do you suppose have been swallowed up by the ocean without a trace? At least these thirty-two made the news for their efforts. Altruism is a luxury you have to be able to afford to dabble in. Look at poor Regis. All he wants to do is complete his education and then go back and fill and pull teeth in his country. Now he is forced to go begging."

My voice was raised, and I was talking to her as if the boat tragedy were her fault. I knew I was being unfair to her: since she was Egyptian, she was not to be blamed for our national hypocrisy. What I was really angry about was her persistent optimism that all things would work out for the good.

We had reviewed our data and re-interviewed our surviving patients in response to our critics and discovered that indeed a small minority of the Haitian men had had homosexual experiences. This fact was seized on by our critics, who ignored the fact that in most of our men, and all of our women, there were still no reports of homosexuality. New theories appeared in the newspapers every day: AIDS started in New York, transmitted by gays vacationing in Haiti to destitute Haitian men forced to prostitute themselves. Conversely, it was said AIDS originated in Haiti as a tropical disease and then was transmitted to vacationing gays by the same mechanism. Or AIDS started in Africa, brought to the Caribbean by Cuban troops returning from Angola, and then was transmitted to the gay community. Again, there were no hard facts to support any of these theories.

There were five patients with AIDS on my ward team at that time (early 1984) , including Herminio, the first gay man admitted to my service who survived long enough to be followed by me in my office. Herminio probably lived his entire life without anyone, other than his lovers, knowing that he was gay. He was forty-two when he was admitted with Pneumocystis pneumonia. His hair was gray and conservatively cut. He had worked as a doorman at a hotel on the beach, but he could have easily passed for a teacher or bank teller. He was frightened by his illness. Even when he was clearly getting better he would ask us if it was time to "call the florist"–a Cuban expression meaning, "Am I going to die soon?" He lived alone with his mother, and he asked us not to tell her what the matter with him was. After his discharge he did well for a while, a fact he attributed to my personal attention to his case.

For one reason or another, most of the original study group had stopped seeing patients with AIDS. Only Margaret, Gordon, and I continued. Because of my other responsibilities and commitments, I followed the fewest. Many of the gay men Margaret followed had been coming to the office long enough now that their deterioration was painfully apparent. Men who originally appeared healthy were now coming in wheelchairs or with pillows because sitting bone they were so wasted on a plastic seat without a cushion of flesh, for too long was unbearable. Many now looked like old men, with sparse white hair, wrinkled skin, and mask-like faces. The secretaries in my office were genuinely moved by their suffering. They knew them all by their first names. Frequently they would be admitted to the hospital and then be absent from the office for several weeks. When they returned, they invariably showed signs of deterioration. When the secretaries saw them in this worsened condition, they were shocked and frequently hid in one of our offices and cried. When one of them would pass away, no one would commiserate with Margaret more than they would. Margaret took each death personally and after each would mourn for several days. During these times it was difficult for anyone to talk to her.

At the time we were fortunate to have on staff a compassionate and dedicated social worker named Alina, who always welcomed a new challenge. One day while Regis was sitting in the waiting area, I called her into my office. I asked her if she would be willing to take on what might be a most difficult case. I outlined Regis's illness, his personality, his current difficulties with the INS, and the social problems his illness was causing him. I told her I was beginning to believe there were no solutions to his problems but that he was one of the most extraordinary people I had ever met. At first she was reticent. I knew she had recently been hurt by letting herself get emotionally involved with patients and their frequently insolvable problems. She told me as much and said she would think about it and let me know by the following day. I didn't push. Perhaps she was having a bad day. Before I had finished with Regis on that visit though, she knocked on my door and told me she would accept my offer and try to help.

When I introduced Regis to Alina, his charm and smile returned for the first time in a good while. She talked with him for an hour. I did not see either of them that day after the interview. The following morning I asked her about her thoughts. She said, "You were right, Art. He is an incredible person."

Soon Alina was talking to Regis almost every day. She managed to get some support for his rent from Catholic Charities, but his situation was rapidly becoming desperate. He admitted that he had not been entirely honest with us about his immigration status. Apparently he had come to this country three years before on a student visa, which had expired.

We sent two letters signed by Margaret, Alina, and myself to the INS explaining Regis's situation and asking that he be allowed to stay in this country for humanitarian reasons. Neither letter was ever formally answered; daily phone calls to the responsible bureaucrats were not returned. Amal prayed with Regis while he waited to see me. In the privacy of the examining room, Regis told me that he appreciated all that we had done for him, but that he felt the situation was becoming hopeless. He wondered why God had forsaken him. I reminded him that I had promised him during his first admission that I would tell him when I thought the situation was hopeless and that I didn't think we had reached that point yet. Although his financial and social problems seemed insurmountable, his T cells were still holding their own. I agreed with him that returning to Haiti would be disastrous, for I was sure there were no resources there to treat his illness. I told him that he had to trust what Alina had said. If there was to be any hope of him remaining in this country he had to go to the INS office and straighten out his immigration status. Then Margaret and I could continue to treat him and Alina could arrange for some financial assistance.

Regis complained of losing vision in his left eye. I tested his vision with our eye chart and found that his vision was still 20/20 in both eyes. His eye examination was normal. He was almost as frightened of blindness as he was of losing his mental powers. I tried to reassure him that his vision tested normally, but he was adamant that his eyesight was failing.

I came to my office one morning and found Alina fighting back tears. My first thought was that she was going to tell me that Regis had died. Instead, she told me the following:

"I'm so angry at myself, Art, for not listening to him," she said, composing herself. "It was exactly what Regis said would happen. For months I have been telling him that he had to go to the INS office and straighten out his immigration status. He told me that if he went there they would arrest him, and I told him that it wouldn't happen, and when he finally took my advice, that's exactly what happened.

"They called me this morning from the emergency room. There are two versions of what happened. Regis claims that he went to the INS office, and after waiting for a long time in line he started not to feel well and asked if he might be moved ahead in line. When the others in line found out he was a Haitian and didn't feel well, someone yelled, 'Hey, you've got AIDS!' Suddenly they were beating him and kicking him until he fell to the ground. Guards came and arrested him and took him to Ward D [our prison medical ward inside the emergency room]. The charges against him were dropped when they found out he had AIDS. Evidently, they didn't want to have to touch him after that.

"The story that the police told the doctors in Ward D was that Regis had tried to cut in line and then began fighting with the others in line and spat at them and told them he had AIDS. He was arrested for disturbing the peace. By the time I got to the emergency room he had disappeared."

I tried to convince Alina that she could not blame herself for the suffering Regis had gone through. We had all heard stories about what it was like at the INS, I told her, but given his situation we had no other choice than to recommend what we recommended.

She wondered out loud why there were two versions of the story. Was there any truth to the police's version of what happened? I told her about the pictures in Regis's album, the ones where he was photographed with the missionaries and the children. Was the person we knew capable of initiating that sort of violence? I had no difficulty deciding which version of the story I would believe.

Regis showed up unexpectedly at our office three days later. Since fleeing the emergency room, he had been living on the streets. He still had bruises on his face and arms from the beating he had received. His clothes were wrinkled and dirty. I told him how sorry I was for all he had gone through. He was very concerned that his vision was now deteriorating rapidly. When I examined him, I found spots on the retina of his left eye, which indicated a viral infection. He had been right about his vision all along. It had just been too early for me to pick up on examination. I spoke with Margaret. There was a possibility that a new antiviral agent might slow or reverse the progression of his blindness. I admitted him to my ward team.

Riding home that evening, Amal and I were somber. I asked her if she believed in the second coming. "As sure as my next breath." she responded.

"And what is prophesied about the Second Coming?" I asked.

"The Book of Revelations says that He will come in a time and in a manner that is least expected." She lowered her eyes in reverence as she always did when she quoted or paraphrased the Bible.

"And what if I told you that Jesus Christ came for his Second Coming as a young Haitian man with AIDS? And what if the entire world missed it? 'Regis, art thou a king?'"

"Don't speak such blasphemy!" she gasped.

"What blasphemy? He may not be crucified but he has certainly been beaten and spat on. Actually, he is being crucified. It's just that it's playing out over three years rather than three hours. If he is not dying for his own sins, he must be dying for ours. Another innocent on the altar. Another virgin in the volcano. You want blasphemy? Not only did you miss the Second Coming, but probably a third, fourth, over a million comings. He comes every time an innocent suffers unto death."

She was silent for a long time. I'm sure she thought that if she provoked me further I would lose my soul forever. Just before I let her off at her home she asked if there were anything she could do. I surprised her by saying, "When he is ready to go home from the hospital, take him home with you."

"Take him home with me?"

"Well, isn't it written, 'and I was naked and you clothed me, and I was starving and you gave me food, and I was homeless and you sheltered me?' You're missing your big chance," I said.

"I would take him home with me if I had a place of my own."

"You have your own room."

The thought of this Egyptian woman taking a Haitian man home to our neighborhood and nursing him back to health was beautiful enough to intrigue me. But I knew that I was kidding myself. And she knew I had won our philosophical war. Such things were just not done. She said nothing further as she got out of the car and entered her house.

17
Sainthood

I ran into my resident, David on my way to rounds the next day. I told him I had admitted one of the patients with AIDS whom I was following.

"Which group of the '4H' club does he belong to?" he asked. According to the house staff, the "4H club" stood for the four groups at risk for AIDS-homosexuals, Haitians, hemophiliacs, and heroin users. I admonished David not to be so cynical, that this patient was special to me. I told him how Regis had worked as a dentist in Haiti, how that was probably how he got his disease, and how we ended up being "blood brothers" as a result of the marmoset experiment. I then told him the circumstances of Regis's admission-how the blindness had been developing and how he had been beaten at the Immigration and Naturalization Service Office.

Regis had spent the night in the emergency room because there were no beds available on the medical service. I had to admit him through the emergency room and declare him life-threateningly ill in order to get him into the hospital, since he could not prove that he was a legal resident of Dade County, Florida. After spending most of the night on a stretcher in the emergency room, Regis was brought to his room on North Wing II. This was the oldest part of the hospital still being used for patient care. It was depressing just to be there. It was darker than the rest of the hospital, the rooms were smaller, and the paint was flaking off the walls, which were colored a hideous green. Regis was deeply depressed and was sure he was not going to leave the hospital. When I approached from the left side, he could not see me. I asked him how he was. He told me he was tired of being constantly asked if he was a homosexual. Evidently, his treatment in the emergency room had not been kind. Something about his mannerisms made me worry he was going to snap under the strain. His hands trembled when he reached for something and when talking to me he would play with his bedclothes or sheets between his fingers and avoid eye contact in a manner that was new for him. I knew how much the blindness frightened him. I asked the house staff to call Ginette, our Haitian-American psychiatry liaison, to ask if she would see Regis for emotional support. Later that day I saw Ginette at a distance down one of the corridors and waved to her. I asked if she had seen Regis yet.

"Oh, I certainly have."

"What did you think?" expecting an outflow of empathy and amazement.

"Unbelievable."

"I know."

"He is a phenomenon."

"Yes, he is," I said, but did not really follow her.

"I mean, I have heard about cases like this, but I've never actually seen one. He really is extraordinary."

"What do you mean?"

"I really don't know quite what the word for it is. It's not quite 'social climber', but he is acting so much out of class. He comes from poor rural Haiti, you know. He would only talk to me in French. He would not talk in Creole, in spite of the fact that I speak Creole fluently. And this business about dentistry by correspondence. He is really trying to make it."

"Ginette, I asked you to see him because he's depressed and suffering. What do you care if he didn't go to Harvard Dental School?"

"Because I think he is lying to you. I think you've been had."

"What do you mean 'had'?"

"I think he is gay."

"Gay! You think that's how he became infected don't you. I've asked him about this over and over. He's a dentist. He leads the life of a saint. The man's a saint!"

"How many saints do you suppose were really gay?"

"Do you have any proof?"

"No, nothing specific, just a feeling. With these sociopathic personalities you can't take anything they tell you at face value."

"Sociopathic!" I almost screamed. "The man spent five years of his life pulling teeth in the backwoods of Haiti. I've seen the pictures."

"You poor bleeding heart," she said. "You idealize everyone. Besides, I've heard of this character from the Haitian community. He is aloof. He takes a superior attitude."

"Ginette, did you do anything to help him?"

"Oh, yes. I was very supportive of him in his struggle against his illness, but I just wanted you to know he's not who you thought he was. I'll continue to visit him daily. Perhaps I can find someone in the community who will take him in."

I left for my office upset but realizing that Ginette's assessment had to be accounted for. After all she could talk with him in his own language and I could not. She knew the culture and I did not... Alina was waiting for me when I got to my office.

"Did you talk with Ginette?"

"Yes, I did. Art, I can't stand it. I can't stand being taken advantage of and lied to."

"How do you know you were lied to?"

"She says he's gay, Art. I believed every word he told me."

"He's one of the few patients with a negative test for syphilis," I responded, weakly.

"She's from his own culture."

"Yes, but I've known him for over two years. He's just a gentle, intelligent man. I've seen the pictures of him performing dental extractions. It was the tainted blood of one of those extractions that infected him. She is a human being just like us and just as likely to be wrong."

"I can't bring myself to go and visit him."

"Because he might be gay or because he might have lied?"

"No. If he were gay I could understand why he might have to lie."

"Look, let's suppose she's right, and he led us down the garden path for all these months. He is still sick, suffering, and destitute. Does it really make any difference? Why do we keep trying to make AIDS someone's fault?"

Although Regis received seven days of a new intravenous antiviral, his vision did not improve. My resident was on my case. He told me that my "blood brother" was trying to use the hospital as a hotel and that I had to help get him discharged. I talked with Regis privately and told him that there was little else I could do for him. I asked him to investigate all of his resources and see if he couldn't find someone he could go home with. He told me he had no one. Reluctantly I told him that perhaps it was time to think about returning to his family in Haiti. At least they could give him food and shelter. He looked at me in despair.

"I came here to succeed," he said. "If I go back, I go back in disgrace. I surely will die."

The next day on rounds Regis told me he had found somebody to go home with. I was surprised by this and didn't quite believe it. I told him I wanted to see him in my office in a week. The house staff had already written his discharge order.

18
Guinea

I examined my own ambivalence toward Regis. I weighed the possibility that he was gay and had lied to us over and over again. There was strong evidence on both sides of the argument. Ginette was a good psychiatrist, and his homosexuality would explain much of his mystery. It played to my personal first principle of psychiatry: Things are never what they seem. On the other hand, I usually know when someone's lying to me. I was willing to grant that he was proud and striving to achieve more than he was born into. This just made him more inherently noble. He could be forgiven the sin of aloofness. But there had never been anything but honesty in his relationship with me. When I had doubted his assessment of what would happen if he went to the Immigration and Naturalization Service, I had been wrong. When I had doubted his blindness, I had been wrong. If I doubted him now, I was at least as likely to be wrong again.

Either way really made no difference. Operationally things were the same. He did not deserve persecution. The death sentence had already been passed. There was no way I was ever going to know for sure. And why did he need to have gotten AIDS from being a dentist and not from being gay for me to like him so much? This last thought was too unsettling for me to dwell on at length on any single occasion, but it haunted me for several years. Perhaps I was not as free of fears, phobias, or prejudices as I wanted to think I was.

For the most part I was depressed that Regis's last hospital admission had been such a failure. He left with even worse vision than he came in with. His long-term prospects for staying in the United States or surviving until we had some sort of treatment were as remote as ever. And a seed of doubt about his honesty had been planted in the minds of the only people in this country who cared about him.

Alina also had resolved her ambivalence. Although we never discussed it, I'm sure her thought process was similar to mine. She became worried when we did not hear from Regis. It was possible that he was living on the streets again. The friend he went home with might not have existed. We were both concerned that the breach of trust from the last admission might keep him from coming back. Why did we ever question his honesty? A week passed.

He came to the office only one more time. I was not there, but he spoke with Alina. He told her he had decided to return to Haiti. Alina made arrangements with the Catholic Charities to pay for his airfare back to Haiti and put him up in a hotel for a few nights. He would be leaving in a few days. As she told me of the plans for his departure her eyes welled up with tears, and I had a terrible lump in my throat.

"He told me that he wanted to thank you for all that you did for him. He said that perhaps if he gets better he will return and complete his education." I told her that I had no delusions. Once he got on the airplane neither of us would ever see him again. She said she was meeting him at the airport and asked if I would like to come.

I looked at my appointment book. Since I was on the hospital wards in the morning and had private patients scheduled in the afternoon, it really wasn't possible. Yet I couldn't help feeling relieved telling her I could not go. It was a precedent I did not want to establish. I cared about Regis. I felt a loss in his leaving and a failure in not being able to do more for him, but I had to keep my distance. It was the only thing protecting me from the pain I saw Margaret experience with each death.

Still, I regretted that I did not have one more chance to see him.

Alina met Regis at the airport as she had promised. She sat with him and waited until the time of departure. He was wearing his three-piece suit again. Her description of his departure sounded like one of those newspaper accounts of a prisoner going to the electric chair. I was even more relieved that I hadn't gone with her. Evidently somewhere during the days since his discharge Regis had regained his composure. She told me he was calm and seemed resigned. Once again, he thanked her for all that she had done for him and asked her to thank me one more time. He pressed her hand, smiled, and then boarded the airplane alone. I knew it would be only a brief stop in Haiti. In voodoo cosmology the souls of the dead are guided by a mermaid, La Sirène, under the sea back to Guinea, their ancestral homeland, the Haitian equivalent of paradise. La Sirene would find Regis.

19
Numb

The numbers of AIDS patients I was caring for and the overwhelming nature of their problems were beginning to numb me. This was particularly true for the Haitian patients, in whom I saw the same cycle: AIDS led to loss of work, which led to enormous social and economic problems and ultimately to death. Although I could talk to them only through a translator, and although I could do precious little to treat their illness or help with their social problems, they continued to smile and thank me after each visit. In terms of sheer numbers, however, the Haitians were decreasing while the numbers of gays and drug users were exploding. It seemed the epidemic was evolving out of control. Every time we figured out a piece of the puzzle it changed into a whole new puzzle.

I can no longer remember the details of each case. Usually, when someone missed an appointment, it meant they had been hospitalized or, worse, had died. Each Thursday some of the patients who came to the clinic were sick enough to require immediate hospital admission. The house staff began to dread being on call on Thursdays. AIDS had intruded into my daily life more than I could have imagined. The phone rang and awoke me from sleep all too frequently, with calls from sick or anxious patients. Real and imagined problems surfaced daily. Even during breakfast, as I sipped my coffee and read the newspaper, I recognized an alarming number of names in the obituaries.

Ten years after the first reported cases of AIDS was approaching, my hopes for a cure had proven naive. All of my early patients had been dead for some time. There were few reminders of those days, really. My career took unexpected turns, taking me first away from AIDS patients and then back with a vengeance. Due to a visa problem, Amal returned to Egypt. When she left, she wished me a thousand blessings. Each blessing turned into another patient with AIDS.

The house staff quietly fulfilled their responsibilities towards AIDS patients but with no enthusiasm and occasional hostility. The specter of contagion haunted my profession. Most physicians wanted all patients tested. Medical students, in particular, seemed torn by the attitudes reflected in the media and what they were taught by their professors. Each year fewer undergraduates were choosing medicine as a career. The most commonly quoted reason: fear of AIDS.

I found an unexpected few moments to speak with Margaret at a meeting in Seattle. We both smiled ironically knowing that we had to travel across the continent in order to have the opportunity to talk to each other. We never saw each other at the medical center those days. Margaret had become an AIDS specialist. No, more than a specialist, an authority. She had conducted the clinical trials that led to the introduction of Zidovudine (AZT), the first medicine found to be partially effective against the AIDS virus, in 1987. She was giving a talk to the meeting about her work. . In a quiet moment before she spoke, she told me that the World Health Organization predicted that by the year 2000 there would be 5 million babies dead from AIDS, 10 million children orphaned, and 15 million dead adults.

"What we have is a pandemic. It will be followed by a second pandemic of drug-resistant tuberculosis. We've not seen anything like this since the Black Death of the 14th century."

"So if there will be twenty million dead, and fifty million people infected with the virus for every one with symptoms of the disease," I said, doing a quick calculation in my head that makes something like a billion infected people by the turn of the 21st century."

These numbers were greater than I could comprehend.

"How many AIDS patients do you think one doctor can care for?" I asked her. "It's exhausting work."

"Five or six hundred at best," she replied.

"So we need a city of doctors worldwide fulltime to care for all these patients. There is no way the medical profession can make that kind of response."

The image of poor people in Africa, Asia, and, of course, Haiti dying with no medical care overwhelmed me. My suspicion that AIDS was somehow differentially preying on the poor had been growing during the late 1980s and early 1990s. Actually, that suspicion had been there initially with our earliest Haitian patients. We had looked at income as a risk factor. Our Haitian patients with AIDS were no poorer than those without AIDS. In retrospect, we had committed a major statistical blunder. The control group should have been a group of rich patients, not other poor people. So for several years, I went against my instincts and tried to find some other link between my Haitian patients and AIDS.

20
Jackie's Story

In 1988, Alina, our staff social worker, persuaded me to help with one of her growing passions–bringing health care to the homeless. I think it might have been a kind of payback for me getting her involved with Regis. At any rate, the social upheavals of the 1980s–the flood of immigrants from Cuba during the Mariel boatlift, many of whom had problems with mental illness----coupled with recession and the impact of crack cocaine on poor communities, had swollen the ranks of Miami's homeless to more than eight thousand. They lived in encampments in the city's parks and under the freeways that crisscrossed the city. As I got more involved, I learned that AIDS had become a huge problem among the homeless.

The clinic was known as the Camillus Health Concern. It was located in an older building of vaguely mission architecture. The skyscrapers of downtown Miami were easily visible from the front door. If the building were one story higher, you could see Biscayne Bay and the cruise ships lined up at the port of Miami four blocks to the east. The immediate neighborhood was surrounded by vacant warehouses, abandoned buildings, parking lots, and pawnshops. Litter was everywhere. Rats scurried around the parking lot, ignoring their human neighbors. Two blocks to the west was the Miami Arena, home at the time of our professional basketball and hockey teams. The arena was built there in an attempt to revitalize the area. Many of my patients worked intermittently at the arena, parking cars, setting up staging, and assisting with the concessions. Those who couldn't find these kinds of jobs tried washing the windows of cars passing by or just plain panhandling. The city fathers very much wanted to move the shelter and the clinic away from the arena. No other neighborhood in the city, wanted it, though.

Every day the food line stretched for two blocks from the kitchen. Every day, when I arrived at work, there were already fifteen to twenty patients lingering outside the door, even though the clinic would not officially open for another hour. The windows of the clinic were papered with messages to patients:

John Smith, see Joan about your lab tests

Jorge Gonzalez, speak with Wilfredo about your disability claim

Inside, the clinic had a wellused, chaotic look. Boxes of donated medical equipment, supplies, and clothing were piled in corners and corridors. The furnishings of the examining rooms and waiting area had been donated and ranged from the merely old to the archaic. An antique x-ray machine gathered dust in one room of the clinic. We couldn't figure out how to use it. The setting would have been depressing if it were not for the staff of nurses, physician assistants, social workers, and support people who assisted

The clinic was founded by Joe, one of our residents, who started volunteering at the shelter when he wasn't on call. He the courage to go out under the bridges and expressways, encounter the homeless face to face, and invite them into the shelter and makeshift clinic. He was making a name for himself. Alina volunteered to write a federal grant, which allowed the clinic to expand and paid for doctors and staff. She asked me if I would volunteer on Tuesday and Thursday nights. At first I was reluctant—homelessness wasn't one of the issues that I cared most about. But once I started, I actually enjoyed it. There was a core group of medical students who came every night-clearly our most dedicated—and lots of patients with interesting problems. After Joe had some difficulties finding a full-time physician, I suggested I'd be willing to work there if he'd also hire Phil.

Phil looked a lot like Willie Nelson, right down to the ponytail. Professionally, he was an interesting story. A "young Turk" pediatric infectious diseases specialist, he had had a falling out with his chair, resigned from the faculty, and entered private practice. He made a lot of money, sold the practice, sailed for two years around the Caribbean, and started to volunteer at the clinic during a refitting layover in port. His volunteering soon became a full-time job—the only job he ever loved, he later claimed. His trademark was a hug. He hugged patients, staff and medical students—"an equal opportunity hugger," he used to say. The students were soon voting him "best teacher" annually. His gentleness with patients was balanced by his intellect and, when necessary, his acerbic wit.

Phil and I could work as a team and bring in medical students to work with us during their primary care clerkships and as evening volunteers. I had received a large grant to move primary care education into the community, and Camillus Health Concern seemed a good place to start. Moving my office into the clinic was a radical move for a tenured professor. I told Margaret I'd have to give up my sessions in special immunology. She and I had been the only ones of the original group left. In truth, I was no longer needed. Her research grants allowed her to fund several new faculty positions, all specializing in AIDS.

We had ten thousand charts in the clinic. Each chart represented a patient who had been seen at least once, a life that had fallen through the cracks of society. Some, like Jennifer, were mentally ill or severely addicted to alcohol or crack cocaine. Others were merely poor or were the victims of bad luck.

The patients coming to the clinic reflected Miami's diversity—black, white, multiethnic, Latino—with one notable exception: There were very few Haitians. In fact, in the six years I worked at the clinic, I had only two Haitian homeless patients. One was a lawyer with bipolar disorder who was too proud to tell his family that he had lost his job. Instead, he just disappeared into the streets. The other had AIDS but didn't want his family to know. I asked the social workers at the clinic how they might explain this. After all, Little Haiti was by far Miami's poorest community. Their consensus: First, there was a very low incidence of alcoholism and drug use among Haitians. It wasn't just that they couldn't afford them alcohol or drugs; their culture didn't condone them. Second, family was the ultimate Haitian safety net. If you fell on hard times, someone in your extended family would always take you in. Finally, as a last resort, returning to Haiti was preferable to life on the streets.

Our biggest success, without a doubt, was Jackie. If ever there was a person who played to all the stereotypes of the AIDS epidemic, it was Jackie—a six foot two, two hundred pound black gay transsexual. "Her breasts are bigger than mine," said Ruth, the clinics head nurse, somewhat jealously.

"It's the estrogen she takes" was my comeback. "If you had that much estrogen flowing through your veins, your breasts would be huge, too."

Jackie was well known to the clinic even before I started working there. She was one of the first patients Ruth had persuaded to be tested for HIV. Not only did she test positive, but her blood counts said she was not far away from full-blown AIDS. She had been living on the streets for years, prostituting herself to support her drug habit—not just the usual crack habit but extraordinary amounts of estrogen, the feminizing hormone. The ultimate outcast and proud of it, she would come to the clinic wearing a blonde wig, a tank top, no bra, the shortest of skirts, and high heels. She was all about attitude. Once I slipped and referred to her as a "he." Her stare was withering. But she needed us. Without estrogen she could not be the woman she wanted to be. I was her only legal source for estrogen. Ironically, in Miami it was getting harder to get estrogen on the street than it was to get crack or heroin.

"Jackie's here to see you, and only you, Art," announced Ruth. "I think she's in love with you."

"Now Ruth—you've just got issues with her cup size."

"Well, it just doesn't seem fair."

In addition to HIV, Jackie had high blood pressure. She adamantly did not want to take AIDS medicines and insisted on taking one and only one medicine for her blood pressure. She knew she was different—I'm sure her attitude was a defense mechanism—but we had leverage: She really wanted estrogen.

"Look, I'm not going to prescribe estrogen to someone who's living on the streets, prostituting herself, maybe infecting others with HIV just because you've got body image issues," I stated, matter of factly, in the semi privacy of an examining cubicle. "On the other hand, I'll meet you halfway. Kick your habit, come in for regular visits, and give up your life on the streets, and we'll work with you."

Jackie was used to bargaining with clients but never about her health. "You would do that for me? I could come here rather than going to the Jackson Clinic? I hate it there. People are always staring." As she said this, she herself was staring down at her own cleavage.

"Sure! Let's get the ball rolling. Start by talking to one of the social workers. We'll get you in a drug program and follow your HIV infection here. You're in luck. Someone actually donated some Premarin to our pharmacy. Who knew? I never thought we'd use it, but why not use it for you?"

I had taken a basic negotiating skill we teach our students—establishing a therapeutic contract—and applied it to a homeless, black, HIV-positive, prostituting transsexual. It worked. She came every month. I knew that in the beginning she came for the estrogen alone, but slowly, surely, she started to take her health seriously. Curiously, her blood counts did not deteriorate appreciably from month to month. It was almost as if she had partial immunity to the effects of the virus. "You'd better watch your blood pressure," I told her during one visit in which she confessed she had been lax about taking her medicine. "Mark my words. Something other than the AIDS virus is going to do you in if you don't take care of yourself."

For every temporary gain or spiritual healing, however, there seemed to be ten medical and spiritual failures. For example, I had to find a way to tell Charisse she would die soon. She and her two children had been living on the street. Her family threw them out when they found out she had AIDS. She felt well, but her T cell count was down to 30. At that level, death is usually just a short time away. "Have you made plans for your children?" I asked when the student medical assigned to her faltered. One of them was with her, a waif under 2, playing with her shoes. He most likely had AIDS also. "You're at a stage of your illness where you will become ill soon. It's time to think about these things." Charisse burst into tears. The student looked as if she might cry also. "No, I haven't made any plans. I'm just going to Hell."

While the clinic thrived, it was also doomed. As a result of the news generated by our Joe's enterprising work among the homeless and the heroic work of our medical students helping victims of Hurricane Andrew in 1992, the University of Miami School of Medicine received the first-ever Community Service Award of the American Association of Medical Colleges. But by the time the award was received, a new clinic administrator had told us of changes mandated by the federal government. The clinic has to reduce losses by enrolling patients in Medicaid and billing our patients for their co-payments. Phil waxed satiric about the absurdity of billing homeless people but the new administrator did not want to hear that. I arranged for Phil to work at another clinic. I departed a few months later.

A week before I left, Jackie came to see me. "I heard you're leaving, Dr. Fournier. Who's going to take care of me?" she asked her hand pressed theatrically to her breastbone.

"There'll still be other doctors here," I responded.

"But they don't know me like you know me," she said. "Inside out, if you know what I mean. What will happen if I don't get my estrogen? I'll just shrivel up and lose all my curves! Listen, I've got an apartment now and insurance – both Medicaid and Ryan White. Can I be your private patient?"

I still had one half day each week during which I saw private patients. I liked Jackie's idea. She would be the one patient I would take with me from the homeless clinic. Managing her problems really was too complicated to turn over to someone else. Besides, we had made a contract and she had kept her end of the bargain. She had kicked her drug habit, was no longer prostituting herself, and was no longer living on the streets.

Jackie kept her appointment. In fact, I followed her in my private practice for twelve years. She came faithfully every month, so that I could follow her HIV infection and renew her estrogen prescription. She was one of the first patients to become a long-term survivor of HIV infection—all told fifteen years without requiring medicines. The office visits became like social calls. She would flirt in an innocent way and socialize with my office staff. When she died in 2004, from health issue not related to AIDS, I was both saddened and relieved. I had been faithful to the end to this most challenging patient.

I viewed leaving Camillus Health Concern with ambivalence. On the one hand, the clinic really had raised the consciousness of Miami concerning its homelessness problems. In a moment of enlightenment, the citizens of Dade County voted to tax themselves to establish a comprehensive approach to homelessness. As a result, the number of homeless people in Miami has been drastically reduced. And we succeeded in giving our students a window on the human condition that few doctors in training ever experience.

On the other hand, with so many social problems drugs, poverty, mental health issues, it was hard to convince myself that the health care services we were developing amounted to much more than a band-aid. I asked myself over and over: Are we making a difference? Could we ever make a difference?

I found the answer in Haiti.

21
Medishare

One Saturday in October 1994, I finished my rounds at the hospital, headed home looking forward to an afternoon of sailing. While changing clothes in my bedroom, I turned on the television to catch the weather forecast. To my surprise, a special event was being broadcast. President Aristide was returning to Haiti. The images alternated between the Little Haiti neighborhood in North Miami, and Port au Prince. I sat down on my bed, arrested by the unfolding spectacle. The plane carrying President Aristide back to Haiti had just landed in the capital. He stepped off the airplane, waving to dignitaries and U.S. troops. When the camera flashed to the presidential palace, tens of thousands of Haitians were outside, awaiting the president's return. Then camera switched to Little Haiti in Miami. Haitian-Americans were dancing in the street. Joy was everywhere.

Back in Haiti, President Aristide entered one of five helicopters that would simultaneously depart for the palace. For security reasons, no one was told which helicopter would land first. I watched as the five helicopters left within a minute of each other for the short trip between the airport and the palace. The crowd outside the palace roared when the helicopters appeared. President Aristide left his helicopter and entered the palace. Several minutes passed, and the cameras focused on the crowds pressing outside the palace fence. The military estimated the crowd at 200,000 people, singing and waving palm fronds. When President Aristide finally stepped in front of the bulletproof glass podium, the crowd exploded with noise and song. The camera flashed back to Miami where Haitian-Americans danced in the street, chanting "TiTid! TiTid!"

I was transfixed by the event. A few hours passed, and I was still sitting on the bed, watching the television. I never went sailing that day. Democracy had come to Haiti.

I had become somewhat acquainted with Haitian politics over the fourteen years I had been caring for Haitian-American patients. That had been a particularly turbulent period in Haiti's history. The decadence of "Baby Doc" Duvalier and his exploitation of the Haitian people ended in 1986 when he fled the country under threat of a popular uprising. He was succeeded by a series of equally undemocratic and repressive military men until 1990 when, to everyone's surprise, a parish priest from Cité Soleil won the first fair election in Haiti's modern history. "TiTid," an affectionate Creole abbreviation that means "little Aristotle," campaigned on the premise that the poor were the overwhelming majority and that it was about time they ran the country. "Peace in the heart, peace in the belly" was his motto. He survived three assassination attempts during the time of the generals. Nine months after his election, the army staged a coup and sent him packing to Venezuela.

American Democrats, particularly key members of the Black Caucus, loved Aristide. Republicans believed his liberation theology was uncomfortably close to communism. Fortunately for Aristide, Bill Clinton was president. In response to the coup, a two-year economic embargo was orchestrated by the United Nations. When that failed to dislodge the junta, an armed intervention led by the United States finally restored Aristide to power. No wonder his return created such a spectacle. For two years the Haitian peasants had endured shortages, price gouging, falling tourism, and the black market, all to get their TiTid back-their leader, perhaps even their savior. And now, thanks to some U.S. Army helicopters, there he was, back in their midst.

At the time, my younger daughter, Suzanne, was in the ninth grade at a private school in Miami. I shared carpool responsibilities with my neighbor, Barth Green, the newly appointed chair of neurosurgery. The following Monday I was passing time with Suzanne in the driveway, waiting for Barth and his two sons. When Barth arrived, rolled down his window, "Do you have any interest in Haiti?" he asked.

"Yes!" I responded immediately.

"Come to a meeting in my office on Wednesday morning. We are going to get into Haiti in a big way."

"Do you mind if I bring some of our Haitian-American faculty?"

"No, bring whoever you want. I've got some doctors from Haiti who are coming up who want to work with us."

"I'll be there," I answered, as I threw Suzanne's book bag into the trunk.

As they drove off, it struck me as odd that Barth would have any interest in Haiti. He had recently started the Miami Project to Cure Paralysis. Surely that must be a full-time job in itself, I thought, not to mention the challenges involved in running one of the medical school's most prestigious departments. I later learned that Barth's good friend from college worked as a missionary in Haiti. His friend's brother was rumored to be the fourth-wealthiest person in Haiti. Barth had asked the family for a sizable donation to his paralysis project. The family complied but with a condition: Barth had to get involved in health care in Haiti.

I arrived at Barth's office ten minutes early the following Wednesday. Three men had arrived before me. One was American. The other two were speaking French. All three were subdued, with somber expressions on their faces, as if they were in church. "You must all be here for the same meeting that I am," I said in French. Danny T. introduced himself in English as the director of a nondenominational Christian missionary group that works in Haiti. Barth's friend from college was his boss.

Marlon and Jerry were twins, distinguishable only by the fact that one had a Shakespearean beard, and the other a goatee. I spoke to them in French, learned from a combination of college classes and a vague recollection of lullabies from my French Canadian grandmother. Upon hearing my French, their expressions changed to broad, relaxed smiles.

"These fine young Haitian doctors want to invite you to come to their country to see what the conditions are there, so that your school can help them," Danny T. explained. It seemed as if he had known them for years. I later learned he had met them for the first time just before I arrived.

Barth was over an hour late, but it mattered little. We were soon joined by Henri, one of our Haitian-American faculty members, and Junia, a Haitian-American student who had worked for me while applying to medical school. Junia was from the same part of Haiti as Marlon and Jerry. With the arrival of these two, the conversation became even more animated and changed into Creole. Marlon and Jerry speak English but were thrilled to have the opportunity to tell their story without the struggle of having to translate it and were delighted to find other Haitians at the meeting. There were times they were speaking so quickly and simultaneously that I couldn't follow what they were saying. Other times, by focusing on the French words I recognized, I could get their meaning. Marlon had trained in obstetrics and gynecology and Jerry in internal medicine. Both, however, spent most of their time performing surgery, since there was a critical shortage of surgeons. The embargo and politics under military rule had left their hospital in ruins. They wanted our help in rebuilding it and an opportunity to come to Miami to learn better operating techniques.

When Barth arrived, the discussion switched back to English. Prior to the embargo, Barth had come up with a plan to provide medical assistance to Haiti with his college friend, but the plan had been put on hold during the embargo.

"The need is even greater now," the twins told us.

Agreement was quickly reached. There was much that our school could do, but the first step would be to put together a team to visit Haiti and assess exactly what the problems were and what we could do about them.

That's how Project Medishare was born. Doing international humanitarian work was not a traditional role for an American medical school, even one that had as strong a tradition of community service as ours. And candidly, our school, as is true of so many medical schools, was struggling to meet the demands for service in Miami. It was hardly in a position to take on the daunting challenges of Haiti. We would need an independent charity to raise funds and support volunteers until we had enough of a track record to compete for government grants and foundation donations. Barth and his college friend chipped in the start-up costs and asked me to put together a team to go down to Haiti and figure out how we could help.

22
Port au Prince

The begging started in the airport parking lot, as we loaded into the small trucks, known as pajeros, which would take us to our hotel. Each of the four small trucks was surrounded by ten to twenty children, mostly boys, ages ranging in age from 8 to 14.

"You got money for me?" "You help me, mister?" "Quarters?" "Dollar?"

These pleas were made softly and frequently with a smile. Our driver responded harshly in Creole but without deterrent effect. We finally began to drive off, with children clutching our open windows, half of them running and half being dragged along with us.

The air was filled with the acrid stench of burning garbage. As we proceeded from the airport to the center of Port au Prince, we could see piles of uncollected trash smoldering by the side of the road. Some of these heaps were taller than me. Some covered a half-acre. Their blue smoke, mingled with the dust blowing off the naked hillsides, stung our eyes and obscured the clear blue sky we had seen from the airplane. Even in the capital, goats were nibbling on trash, live chickens hung by their feet in open-air markets, and burros were used as beasts of burden. For that matter, so were humans. Small men pulling two-wheeled carts piled high with boxes were everywhere. Women carried water, food, or bread on their heads. We passed a military checkpoint on the way downtown.

With that one exception, we saw no sign of law, nor any sign of disorder. The narrow streets were crowded with people. In fact, it seemed as if the entire city lived in the streets. Automobile traffic was heavy and slowed by the crush of people. However, a gentle toot of the horn and pedestrians immediately yielded the right-of-way to the automobiles. There were no traffic lights working, but our drivers were skilled with their horns as they approached intersections or corners and were careful to negotiate the seemingly endless series of potholes, puddles, and ruts. If we stopped our caravan, children appeared from the crowd and asked for money. They were gently discouraged by our drivers. For the most part, though, we were ignored. How strange for such a poor country to have so much industry in its streets. People were weaving hats and baskets from palm fronds, making rattan furniture, and refurbishing old box springs, all out on the streets. Brilliantly colored paintings hung from walls and fences.

"A nation of artists," Henri volunteered, "but who's going to buy their works?"

Most of the traffic consisted of large trucks carrying construction materials or "tap-taps," the vehicles that serve as Haiti's public transportation. Tap-taps, named for the sound made by their engine, ranged from small pickups outfitted with a carved wooden bonnet, to city buses, to twelve-wheelers. For a few gourdes (a coin worth about two U.S. cents) one could travel all around the city on the smaller pickups or, for a few gourdes more, all the way to Cap Haitien or Jérémie. The larger tap-taps had their routes painted on the side, front, and back. They were decorated with bright colors, paintings, designs, and frequently hand-carved wood trim. They also had elegantly painted religious phrases or pawòl granmoun, expressions of folk wisdom. Most spewed out diesel smoke that mingled with the smoke from the piles of burning garbage to sting our eyes and make us pinch our nostrils. It seems there had been no trash pickup during the three years of the embargo. People burned their garbage with gasoline or kerosene when the piles became insurmountable obstacles.

The color of the streets varied from drab concrete gray to explosions of bright colors, particularly around the open-air markets, with a seeming abundance of squash and vegetables accented by the white feathers and red combs of the upside-down chickens. In most places the sidewalks thronged five to six people deep, all of whom seemed to have some place to go or something to do. Toothless old people mingled with groups of school children in uniforms wearing backpacks

We stopped at the Holiday Inn before going to the university hospital. In the back of the hotel was a courtyard, a tropical garden with shade, a breeze, and leaves that seemed to soak up the haze, dust, and diesel smoke. Those of us who were in Haiti for the first time shared our initial impressions. For our Haitian-American faculty, it was the beginning of a four-day reunion. Some had not been home for more than a decade, and none had been able to return home during the three years of the embargo. Every new face in the hotel came over and introduced himself or herself, followed by smiles and embraces.

Marlon and Jerry rejoined us. They would be inseparable from us over the next four days. They were in their element now. Any shyness that afflicted them in Miami had melted away in their own country. They were ecstatic that we had come and hopeful that we could help them and their people, even if that prospect for help was in the distant future. They were classic twin brothers. One started a sentence and the other finished it. Their English was excellent when they were fresh, but when they were tired they sometimes struggled for words. They were kind enough to use English, since most of our group did not speak French or Creole. They carried small radiophones, which were constantly ringing, and they had the uncanny ability to carry on one conversation concerning patient care in Creole with each other while speaking to us in English. Their energy was boundless and their dedication obvious. They wanted to take us on a tour of the university hospital before the officially planned tour the following morning. As we passed by a nursing class, several students waved, called their names, and blew kisses.

The university hospital had been built by the U.S. Marines during their occupation in the first half of the 20th century. It reminded me of the hospital in which I had done my residency two decades ago--a complex of two-and three-story buildings with barrel-tile roofs and open-air porches. Across the street from the entrance to the hospital were a collection of drugstores, mortuaries, and coffin makers.

As we were entering the emergency area, we passed two older Toyota vans with red crosses painted on their sides. One had its hood raised, and the other had a flat tire. "Our ambulance fleet," commented Marlon dryly. Between the two defunct ambulances and the small door labeled "Emergency" was a tap-tap with two legs dangling outside. The woman inside had had a seizure and had yet to regain consciousness. She was being tended to by her fellow passengers. We entered a dark corridor. The walls were painted a dinghy olive drab, and the stale smell of urine permeated the air.

"This is the ER stabilization area." The room we were in had several small cubicles. In one a resident was quietly suturing a laceration. In another cubicle a two-day-old baby with a colectomy was nestled in a crib with his mother at his side. Jerry explained that the baby was born with an imperforate anus. He and his brother had performed a colostomy to save the baby's life.

We proceeded through a maze of dimly lit corridors and passageways connecting one ward to the next. Each ward contained twenty to thirty beds. They were divided according to services-medicine, orthopedics, surgery, pediatrics, and obstetrics. Each ward had more patients than there were beds. On most wards this meant that patients were doubled-up, two per bed. One the orthopedics ward, though, because of traction and other hardware requirements, there was only one patient per bed. The mattresses on the beds were old and stained. There were rarely sheets. There were no nurses, no toilets, no running water, and no medicines. Marlon explained that if they wanted a patient to have medicine, they had to write the patient a prescription, and either the patient or a family member would have to take it to a pharmacy across the street and return with the medicine to the hospital. At this point the patients were responsible for taking it themselves. Food and nursing care were provided by families. Those patients without families depended on passersby or fellow patients.

Flies were everywhere in the surgical ward, where burn victims were recuperating. Burns are common in Haiti, where most people cook over open fires. Children frequently burn themselves when they pull over pots of food suspended over the fires by tripods. The burn victims avoided the flies by sleeping under mosquito netting. There were probably six or seven burn victims there that day, their dark uninjured skin in sharp contrast to the pink, yellow, and mottled burned tissue. Flies buzzed around a container filled with antiseptic solution. Jerry described how, without a sterilizer, unsterile gauze pads were dipped into the antiseptic solution to pack the wounds of surgical patients. Eighty percent of the emergency surgical patients developed sepsis, and sixty percent died. Many patients seemed to be there because they had no place else to go. Their doctors could figure out they had some terrible malady, but they had no medicines to treat it.

Our next stop was an orphanage in a place called Post Cazeau, a complex of newer buildings on a large plot of land, near the airport. We could see planes taking off and landing just beyond the treetops. Marlon and Jerry said they would like to build a new hospital in a vacant field next to the orphanage some day. Miriam, the director, volunteered that she would donate the land. She also had land out in the countryside, in a village called Pestel due west of Port au Prince, that she would donate to Project Medishare.

Miriam trained as a nurse and has been doing missionary work in Haiti for twenty-three years. In addition to running the orphanage, her organization, World Harvest, sponsored open-air clinics in villages in the countryside.

"As bad as things are in Port au Prince, they're ten times worse in the countryside," she informed us. "When we hold one of our clinics, two to three hundred people will come from all around. Children with malnutrition and typhoid fever, people with tuberculosis and malaria. In Pestel there are 60,000 people in the surrounding area and not one doctor. The government has a building there, but there's no one to staff it. We're so pleased you're going to help."

Miriam, her staff, and the orphans set up tables in a field next to the orphanage, under a canopy of palm fronds to provide needed shade. Our Haitian hosts were in agreement with regard to their priorities. First, the university hospital needed to be resuscitated as a teaching hospital. Then it needed to train doctors and nurse practitioners who could provide general medical care. Finally, there needed to be a coordinated system for transportation around the country and a way to maintain medical equipment and supplies. Project Medishare, representing, at least in the Haitians' eyes, the University of Miami School of Medicine, could help in all areas–by donating medical equipment and supplies, by developing the training that was needed, and, of course, by raising money.

As a group of teenagers played homemade instruments and sang Haitian folk songs under a tree the entire afternoon, Miriam provided lunch and a tour of the orphanage. The orphans sang songs and presented Barth with a bouquet of flowers in honor of our visit. Miriam told us the story of each orphan in the chorus. Most were survivors of the wreck of the Neptune, a ferry boat from Jérémie that capsized during a storm in February 1993 resulting in the drowning of more than nine hundred people. While the incident received fleeting coverage in the American press, it had become legendary in Haiti. Every street artist had a painting of the wreck of the Neptune, full of visual imagery of drowning innocents.

The children, some sixty all told, were well behaved and affectionate. They made friends with every member of the group. Miriam told us that each one was hoping for adoption. Most of the faculty completed the tour with a child holding on to each hand. I had been warned by some Haitian friends in Miami to beware of the missionaries. Many missionaries are seen by the Haitian people as agents of the Center Intelligence Agency, and some missionaries have come to Haiti with pejorative attitudes about voodoo or the Haitian work ethic. Much of the ceremony at the orphanage would have struck a cynic or skeptic as a calculated play for sympathy, but I felt skepticism draining from me in the face of such obvious need.

We reentered our Pajeros and snaked slowly in silence up the hill to Petionville, where our hotel was located. Although it was late at night, the life in the streets still pulsed. Although Petionville is considered a well-to-do suburb, there were people begging on the street outside our hotel. Parked immediately next to the hotel was an abandoned hulk of a burned-out car, with five children living in it. Several members of our team kept bringing food from our meals out to the children. The hotel itself, built in Caribbean gingerbread style during a brief surge in tourism in the 1970s, was an oasis of comfort and service. This only served to further subdue the group. Some were too emotionally moved after the experiences of the day to enjoy the hotel's hospitality. Others went directly to the bar.

I could see that social class was a huge issue in Haiti. I had read about this unique part of Haiti's history as I prepared for our trip. The French plantation owners of Saint Dominique were true aristocrats–counts and marquis'–but only French men were willing to give up the luxuries of France and endure the hardships and risks of the tropics. So they took slaves as concubines. The progeny of these liaisons were treated by their fathers as a special class. They weren't free, but their fathers acknowledged their paternity and allowed them to own land, receive an education, and manage the plantations. So the Haitian revolution was really two revolutions rolled into one–a slave uprising by Africans, taking advantage of the chaos created by the French revolution to win their freedom, and an Oedipal revolt by the lighter-skinned mulattes. Both classes joined forces to drive out the French. Shortly thereafter, however, conflicting visions of who owned the country erupted into civil war. The result was a stalemate, with the Africans and their descendants controlling the land in the countryside and the mullates controlling the institutions – government, church, and education. The mulattes became, in effect, an unlanded aristocracy. Class politics became an endless cycle of power plays, oppression, and revenge.

These class tensions have dominated the history of Haiti since the revolution-one class believing that Haiti is their birthright, the other that only they have the knowledge and skills to manage the country. Both are simultaneously dependent on and suspicious of the other. These tensions were readily apparent at the bar at the Kinam Hotel. The staff, coal black, talked among themselves in Creole, but responded to their patrons in French. The bar clientele were all light skinned, fashionably dressed, and insistent on impeccable service. Their eloquent Parisian French shamed my French-Canadian patois.

I pulled Michel, one of my Haitian-American colleagues, aside to a quiet corner and asked him, "What's the attitude of the elite to the poor here?"

Michel himself is a very light-skinned Haitian but more of a member of the intellectual elite rather than the economic elite. He traced part of his ancestry to French Huguenots from Nantes, and in truth the only hint of Africa in his features is the black curliness of his hair. He showed me on a map of Haiti where the plantation bearing his ancestral name was located. However, Michel was the rare individual with the ability to step outside class and take a truly objective view

"I'd have to say, there's a spectrum of attitudes that range from 'noblesse oblige' to 'let them eat cake'. You can live well in Haiti, even if you're not particularly rich, if you come from the right family. The poor provide servants—cooks, maids, and chauffeurs. Some are treated as members of the family; others are frankly abused. I've always found it ironic that a country born of the only successful slave revolt in the world has so many of its people working as servants. For them it's almost like the revolution never happened. For the most part, however, most of the elite are ignorant of the plight of the poor. They're isolated from the problem. They never leave the capital."

"The gulf between the rich and poor is pretty glaring," I remarked. "The houses on the crest of the hill above the hotel are as impressive as anything in Miami and with a much better view. Isn't it a little ironic that we're down here trying to help and some of the elite could care less?" I asked.

"It's not that simple, Art," Michel responded. "Some do care. Charity is different here, however. A family might quietly support a poor family they know or one particular orphanage. Occasionally, a prominent family will adopt a cause like a hospital or an orphanage. Most of the doctors are sons or daughters of the elite, and all of us give back to a greater or lesser extent. Look at Marlon and Jerry. The thing is you're seeing all this with the eyes of an American. I wonder really if it's all that different in the United States, except there's more wealth and less poverty there. But take everything we've talked about with regard to "class" and substitute "race," and that's what you've got in the States. How many white Americans feel any responsibility or sense any connectedness to black Americans?"

23
Cité Soleil (Sun City)

The following morning we returned to the university hospital for the official visit. I spoke with our Haitian-American faculty as we assembled outside prior to the tour. All three were stunned by what they had seen the previous day. "Haiti always was a poor country, but the health care system worked," said Michel. "I trained here in medicine. I had a good experience. Now, there is nothing left. It's like a shell."

The newly appointed director of the hospital introduced us to several members of the faculty and medical staff. He was quite candid. "We have nothing!" We formed a caravan of cars and head for Cité Soleil. Ten minutes later, we took a left turn. The narrow road dropped 10 feet in elevation, flattened out, and plunged straight ahead into a seemingly endless plain of cardboard and tin shacks. Footpaths snaked between the shacks, and wisps of smoke rose from the open fires used for cooking. The smell of urine and feces intermingled with smoke and the aroma of cinnamon and vanilla. There was even more life in the streets - buying, selling, sidewalk industry than in Port au Prince. People wearing rags and naked children bathing in washbasins or chasing each other between the shanties mixed with people in starched white shirts, lace-trimmed dresses, or school uniforms.

The only other motorized vehicles on the road were trucks and Caterpillars hauling out piles of garbage. The government had made Cité

Soleil its first priority for garbage removal. "How silly," I thought, since the whole encampment was built on a pile of mud, rocks, puddles, and trash. Whenever the process of trash removal slowed our progress, children again surrounded us, gently asking for money. The adults occasionally smiled and waved but, in general, paid no attention to us, as if it would be impolite to stare at such strange people in such strange vehicles. Although human voices sounded everywhere, without the noise of the automobiles, there seemed a strange aura of peace in Cité Soleil.

It was even quieter in St. Catherine's Hospital, which rests behind a wall in an enclosure that includes a school and an orphanage. It's located in the further reaches of Cité Soleil, a short distance from Port au Prince harbor. From the second story of the maternity ward, we could see children playing and women washing their clothes in a sewer lake the size of a football field. In fact, one can see all of Cité Soleil from that vantage point, a tribute to its flatness, the low height of its huts, and the compactness of the area, home to 200,000 people.

St. Catherine's was run by a private group under contract with the Catholic Church. Compared to the university hospital, it was functional. Here, there were nurses in the wards, clean sheets on the beds, and a food service. Most touching was the maternity ward. Most births in Haiti take place at home, but conditions in Cité Soleil were so unhealthy that St. Catherine's promoted "intensive" prenatal care and in-hospital delivery. There was still crowding, with two mothers in each bed, 60 mothers all told, along with their newborns. In St. Catherine's the newborn child was kept with its mother, who nursed it as needed. I was struck with the contrast to our nurseries in the United States, with their plastic bassinets, confining blankets, and bottles of formula. "Why should a newborn spend the first days of its life mostly in isolation?" I thought. Three sets of twins were born the day we were there. One set was nursing simultaneously, one on each of their mother's breasts. Perhaps there were things we would learn from Haiti, despite its problems, rather than assuming that coming from the United States we knew it all.

"This is better. Don't you think?" I said to Ruth, the nurse from Miami's homeless clinic, as we were leaving. Touring St. Catherine's, I didn't notice that she had dropped out of the tour in the maternity ward or that she had been crying.

"Better?" She whispered incredulously. "What hope for life could these children possibly have? You saw what we drove through to get here. They'll stay in the hospital for two days and then go home to what? A dirt floor, a cardboard roof, and an open fire? It's so sad. They have nothing."

I invited Ruth to join the team because I hoped her experience running the homeless clinic in Miami would translate into practical advice as to how to address primary care and nursing issues in Haiti. Based on our working together at Camillus Health Concern, I knew I could count on her for no-nonsense answers.

"They have their mothers' love, and their fathers', too." My words convinced myself, but I'm not sure they convinced Ruth.

"Get real, Art," she came back at me. "This is one notch above hopeless."

That afternoon, on the way back to the hotel, our caravan ventured down one of the few paved side streets in Cité Soleil. The Pajeros stopped so that the journalists from the Herald and Channel 10 could take pictures of children playing in the open drainage. There was not a tree or a blade of grass in Cité Soleil, only people, animals, shacks, and trash. Our vans were surrounded by 30 to 40 children, laughing, smiling, begging, and reaching through the open window to touch us.

I spoke my first words in Creole: *"Nou pa genyen lajan"* ("We don't have any money").

"W'ap ban mwen valiz-la?" ("You give me your purse?")

The words, almost sung in a sweet soft voice, came with a smile from a young girl with an angelic face. She pointed to Ruth's pocketbook wedged between us.

"She'd like your pocketbook, or its contents," I translated. I was just starting to crack the code between French and Creole.

"Ou trè bel" ("You are very pretty").

"Mèsi, msye" ("Thank you, sir").

"Kijan ou rele?" ("What's your name?").

"Regine, msye" ("Regine, sir").

When she realized we wouldn't give her the purse, she became content to stroke Ruth's dress and leg with her extended finger. She appeared about twelve, her budding breasts partially exposed by her tattered T-shirt. Her companions on my side of the car asked for the four Dixie Cups we had used for drinking water and that were kept in the back of the van. When I gave them the cups, the lucky four ran off to play with them in the drainage, followed by an envious entourage. Regine and several others stayed with us. I wondered how many other strangers she had begged from. How unreal to be sitting in the middle of Cité Soleil, surrounded by 200,000 of the poorest people I had ever seen.

I had more money in my wallet than any of these children's parents (if they had parents) earned in a year-maybe 10 years. And yet there was no sense of danger. In fact, there was a mystifying aura of peace, fostered by the absence of cars and the softness of the children's voices. Then a dark thought entered my mind. Anyone who wanted to could take advantage of these children. Any one of them, boy or girl, could probably be had for as little as a quarter.

I thought back to our article about AIDS among Haitians and the controversy it had generated. While our critics were wrong in claiming that our patients were all gay, perhaps there was a grain of truth in the assertion that gay men had been coming to Haiti and giving money to young boys for sexual favors. It probably was not just a gay thing, though. There were probably plenty of straight men making the short flights from Miami or New York to buy sex from Haitian girls and women. Exploitation has no sexual orientation. There had never been much debate in the medical journals or the press as to whether the virus evolved in the United States and was transmitted here or vice versa, or in some entirely different place (we now know it probably originated in Africa). But seeing Cité Soleil, I could only wonder what the point of the debate was. Wasn't it just another way of fixing blame? There had already been too much blame, I suddenly realized and not enough understanding. If anything, it was politics, economics, and exploitation that spread the virus. For that we're all responsible and we're all to blame. The majority just loves to pin the blame on a minority, particularly one that can't fight back.

As I sat in the van, surrounded by squalor, another thought struck me.

"My God, we've created the world's largest Petri dish,"

The desolate setting was ideal for growing genetic material, human, viral, and bacterial. The temperature, at ninety degrees, was heating up the water seeping through the garbage. Children and adults were washing, drinking, and excreting this water, sometimes with cuts or open sores on their feet. In this soup of human and non-human DNA, anything could evolve. AIDS could have started here, or in Lagos, or perhaps in Bangkok. It didn't matter where it started. Poverty was the issue, not sex, and we could do something about that.

Regine had finishing running her finger across Ruth's leg. I thought of my own daughters. What accident of birth or stroke of fate destined them to a life of comfort in Miami and Regine to be begging and perhaps prostituting herself to strangers in Cité Soleil?

"Wake up," I told myself. "You can do something about this!"

That night, back at the hotel, I allowed myself the luxury of a bottle of wine after dinner. I sat on the terrace sharing the day's events with the Haitian-Americans in our group-Michel, Henri, Ron, and Junia. I discovered we all shared the blessings of a Catholic education: a broad base of philosophy, theology, and history, with the church's particular spin. My education and Junia's, guided by the Augustinian fathers in the United States, had emphasized philosophy and theology. Michel, Henri, and Ron, taught by the Jesuit fathers in Haiti, were strong in history, language, and politics.

Michel could speak both Latin and Greek. He laughed at how hard he had studied those subjects for so many years. "What relevance do Latin and Greek have to life in Haiti?" he asked. "But the good fathers believed we needed a classical education."

Junia mentioned how hard it was going to school in Miami. Her parents had immigrated so that their children could get an education. Her schoolmates teased her relentlessly about her language and her clothes. All lamented how many traditional values were lost in the process of Americanization.

I confessed my role in the Haitian AIDS study. They all looked at me with expressions that said, "Art, how you could have done such a thing?" Unfortunately, the study was infamous. I realized that all my colleagues had experienced the unspoken accusation—"You're Haitian. You must have AIDS"—and I was partly responsible for that. I realized the absurdity of lumping all Haitians together. Here was Michel, light-skinned progeny of professional-class parents, sitting beside Junia, coal dark, whose father died when she was young and whose mother worked as a custodian. And then there was Regis, my "blood brother" dentist, and Regine, the young girl in Cité Soleil. What did they have in common? Yes, they were all Haitian, but that was about all they had in common. So why would being Haitian, per se, put you at risk for an infectious disease? How naive we had been.

24
Lost

I awoke that morning at four o'clock. My mind was full of images and ideas, visions of the people in Cité Soleil and the hospitals and plans of how we could help. Not wishing to disturb my roommate Lynn, I silently slipped outside the room and went to the pool to recline on a chaise lounge. The people who had been sitting around the terrace a few hours earlier had completely disappeared, some to their rooms and some to dance through the night. The night staff at the hotel had curled up on couches and were fast asleep. There was no electrical power in Petionville that night or, for that matter, in much of the rest of Haiti. Since the United Nations-sponsored embargo to restore Aristide, the capital averaged four hours of electricity each day. As a result, the stars were brilliant and plentiful in the clear skies above. It was a surprisingly cool evening, with a gentle breeze and no mosquitoes.

The tranquility ended with the sound of voices singing in the street. Why would people be singing at 4:00 in the morning? I asked myself. To see over the wall that protected the hotel terrace from the street, I had to climb the stairs to the second-story balcony. Coming up the hillside street next to the hotel was a group of five women, all balancing twenty-gallon buckets of water on their heads. One woman would sing a line, and the other four would respond in chorus. It was a happy, joyous song, like gospel music, except in Creole rather than English. Earlier in our trip I had noticed the head wraps-the torquettes-all the women in Haiti wore. They were suggestive of turbans, and the group coming up the hill demonstrated to me their purpose: It made it easier to balance heavy loads on their heads. I thought back to Jeanette and her seminar on voodoo and the zombie curse. Now it was becoming clear, as I listened to the women singing. Here the French god and the older African gods lived side by side, but the old gods were closer to the people and maybe even more helpful to them.

At 4:30 the roosters began to crow. Oddly, this reminded me of home, since I lived within earshot of Little Haiti and always arose early. At 5:00, the church bells began ringing and the scent of freshly brewed Haitian coffee permeated the air. It was Sunday. I had lost track of time. I decided to leave the hotel to watch the sunrise. Even at that hour there already was an old, toothless woman standing just outside the door, begging. To the right, about a block away, a footpath zigzagged up a steep hillside. There was much traffic going both up and down. I wondered where the path might lead, and guessed it might provide me with the best sunrise opportunity.

The path was no more than a yard wide. If you passed someone, you both had to turn sideways. The people coming down the hill were a mixture of families going to church and people carrying water or vegetables to the Petionville open-air market. Many of these people were barefoot. I wished I was barefoot, since the steepness of the path and the slipperiness of my leather soles forced me to frequently use my hands to assist in my ascent. People coming down the path would offer me their hands in assistance. It was hard for many to conceal their bemusement at a blan climbing the path, and yet everyone smiled as we passed and everyone said *"Bonjou."*

"Bonjou," I responded, and returned their smiles.

The top of the path revealed a dirt road that encircled an old stone wall, resembling a fort or castle. The night before, Michel had told me how, after they had expelled the French in 1804, the Haitian leaders built forts and castles in high strategic positions throughout the country, anticipating that the French would return to try to recapture their prize.

The view from the base of the fort was spectacular. I could see the entire city of Port au Prince and the entire valley the city sits in, turning into countryside as it extended to the east. To the north and to the south were long sweeps of coastline with rugged mountains. In the city three things stood out-the presidential palace, the cathedral, and the cemetery. Above the wall the mountains rose perhaps another 2,000 feet, dotted with the homes of some of Haiti's wealthiest families.

The elite had taken a lot of criticism in the American press for its role in supporting the dictatorship. One writer had even coined the phrase "morally repugnant elite," or MRE for short. The attitudes I heard expressed in the hotel bar toward President Aristide—sometimes stated openly, sometimes veiled in political correctness—shocked me. In the American press during the embargo, Aristide was portrayed as a folk hero—a saintly, scholarly man with the courage to stand up to the dictators. Now, in the post intervention politics of both Haiti and the United States, the press at times and the opposition continuously presented a different picture. Aristide was just another demagogue, with his own circle of henchmen and assassins, all out to get rich in the process of controlling the government, a new aristocracy of the formerly poor. What had I gotten myself into? How much of this was true, and how much represented class-based politics? As an American it was best not to pass judgment, at least until I knew more.

Focus on our humanitarian mission. Stick to health care. Don't take sides. Stay out of politics, I reminded myself as I thought back on my experiences of the day before.

Stop trying to lay blame on anyone. Just accept the fact that Haiti is yin and yang—a culture with two sides—one elite, book-educated, light-skinned, Catholic, French, and urban; the other poor, tradition-educated, dark-skinned, voodoo, African, and rural. On my descent down the path, back to the hotel, I extended a helping hand to those ascending, as had been done for me a short while before.

25
Escaping the Curse

On our last day in Haiti, our hosts wanted to take us out of the city. Life in rural Haiti is very different from life in the capital. Our destination was Kenscoff, about fifteen kilometers away, on the other side of the mountains that rim Port au Prince. We ascended quickly from Petionville, through a partially canopied road. Trucks heading in the opposite direction were filled with workers returning from the mountain quarries. In valleys and ravines we could see clusters of huts and the smoke of open-air fires. On the road there was a thin but steady stream of people-women heading to town on burros, or with baskets on their heads, or men herding goats or carrying sheaves of wood. We crested one mountain ridge, descended, then started up again in a new valley we could not see from Port au Prince. The countryside was dotted with small wood-frame homes decorated with wood carvings and palm-thatched roofs. Farmers tilled their fields, and in the distance long lines of women could be seen descending footpaths, carrying produce on their heads. Kenscoff was about three-quarters of the way up the valley, with a deep ravine and terraced slopes on the opposite side running all the way up the mile-high mountain. Just before Kenscoff, there was a Baptist mission, a museum, a clinic, and an orphanage. Across the road was a collection of leather goods and paintings for sale by local artisans.

The museum contained more than I expected. In addition to Arawak pottery and slave-carved furniture, there was a collection of toys artfully constructed from trash by the children of the mission, which is the oldest in Haiti. We met the foundress, who, with her husband, had started the mission and clinic 49 years earlier.

"You see the terraces on the hillside? The mission helped the people build them, so they could farm," explained Danny T.

"Unfortunately, they didn't hold during tropical storm Gordon last summer," the foundress added. "Seven hundred people were washed down the ravine. Some were never found. The saddest thing, though, were those who climbed out, covered with mud, who lost everything. We still have seven families we haven't found homes for. They just live outdoors, foraging for food. If you find someone in the U.S. who wants to do something, we'd appreciate your help."

There was irony in her comments about the flood. There had been a small item in the Miami newspaper about seven hundred people drowning in Port au Prince. Either these people in Kenscoff were totally ignored, or the reporter didn't know the difference between the city and the countryside. As a second irony, that day the news reported that fifteen hundred people died in an earthquake in Japan. That tragedy made front-page news for a week.

We toured the grounds, including the clinic. They used a butcher's scale with an attached sling to weigh the children. The clinic was busy, with a line of people outside the door waiting to be seen. Orphans, identifiable by their shared uniforms, were running around chasing each other. We had lunch in the American-style cafeteria. The menu was mostly hamburgers and hot dogs. I had no interest in eating, but I did order a plate of French fries and sat down with Ruth at a window with a view of the whole valley.

As we were preparing to leave, Henri and Junia gave me books as a gift for making their trip possible. One was a book on learning Creole, and the other was a book of Creole proverbs. The foundress gave me a toy helicopter made of oil containers and bottle caps and a book entitled God Is No Stranger. The text contained spiritual expressions from the people of Haiti. The photos were beautiful-candid, but capturing the souls of their subjects. To my surprise, on the twenty-fourth page was the same woman I had seen in a photo in Regis's book thirteen years before--the one sitting in the chair having her tooth extracted.

This was your mission, wasn't it Regis? It had to be. It was the first, and the only one here long enough for you to grow up in and to return as a dentist. Is this where you returned to die? Are you here in one of the tombs I saw as we ascended the mountain? Or did you feel too stigmatized to return home? Did you die in the hospital in Port au Prince? Are you buried in that huge cemetery I could see from the hillside in Petionville? Is it a comfort that I still think of you? It has been 12 years and not a week goes by that I don't think of you. You and all the others. But especially you, my blood brother. You were infected by the blood of one of your patients. The first occupational fatality. The first to die as a consequence of your professional duties.

You should have been hailed as a hero. Instead, they insisted you were gay, so they could blame you for your fate, wash their hands of your blood. If you were an innocent victim, there might be other innocents as well, and God would have no justice or mercy. But you were all innocent. We have no one to blame but ourselves-our own ignorance and willingness to tolerate intolerable conditions. You were just the most irrefutable case, and it took me years to understand. It's bad enough that you all had to die, but how much did we add to your suffering through stereotype and blame?

You had a curse on you, didn't you? But, then, so did I. Cursed by naiveté and enslaved by conventional thinking. I've been sleepwalking through the biggest medical event in my lifetime, enslaved by the constraints of my world and ignorant of the reality of yours. It took this visit to your home to wake me up. Once you see it, it all makes sense— the poverty and the things some people have to do to survive in places like Cité Soleil. So even if we can't cure AIDS, we ought to be able to do something about its cause. The problem is most of my colleagues have never ever seen anything like this. They're under a zombie curse that's even worse than mine. No point in worrying about that now, though. I've got to focus on what I can do—how I can make a difference, Regis. I promise I'll try.

Ruth caught me staring across the valley, lost in thought. She touched my arm. "Time to go, now," she spoke softly. "What were you thinking about?"

"Just day dreaming. I knew a person from here once. A dentist. He died of AIDS. One of the first." I was still staring across the valley.

"How do you know he was from here?"

"He told me so, in a roundabout way. Are you glad you came to Haiti?"

"Glad?" I said. "It's been the most moving experience of my life."

When it came time to leave, Marlon and Jerry came to the airport to see us off.

"You'll come back, won't you, Dr. Fournier? Come for Carnival."

"Biensur, Marlon et Jerry. *Ayiti meté met yon hounga sou mwen*" ("Haiti cast a spell on me").

I put this phrase together from the book Junia had given me a few hours before. It took Marlon, Jerry, and all the people in our group by surprise, and they broke out in laughter. I needed a laugh myself. It seemed like Haiti had freed me from a zombie curse that had enslaved my mind all these years.

"I must come back," I said.

26
House Calls

The culture shock of returning home to Miami started even before we landed. Out my window I could see row after row of neat suburban houses, most with swimming pools. Sunlight reflected off the windows of the skyscrapers downtown, while cars streaked along the expressways. I was returning from another world.

My wife, Janet, and my daughter Suzanne met me at the airport. As I entered the car, Janet started talking about home issues and things that had transpired in our family while I was gone. I could tell by her body language and facial expressions that she didn't want to bring up the trip, fearing, correctly, that it might have changed our lives forever. She did not like my work in Haiti but would not bring it up, at least not right away. So it was Suzanne who, ten minutes into the trip home, first inquired, "Well, how was it, Dad?"

"Words fail me, Suz," I said, "Imagine a place where you can't even count on clean water or electricity, where the children can't count on going to school. Yet the people were beautiful, and there's so much we can do to help. I'll tell you one thing, though. We're never going to take anything we have here for granted ever again."

Shortly after returning, Barth, Michel, and I set up a meeting with Bernie, dean of the University of Miami School of Medicine to present our plans for helping Haiti. Our students and residents could come as volunteers to orphanages almost immediately. Just doing screening exams and creating medical records would be a huge benefit for those children. We could do health fairs like the ones we do in Key West, only modified for Haitian health issues. We had met many Haitian doctors—Marlon and Jerry, for example—who wanted to come to Miami for further training. Michel was particularly interested in introducing training in family medicine, as this discipline did not exist in Haiti. But to accomplish any of this, we would need the dean's blessing.

Bernie had been the dean for my entire tenure on the faculty. He had been instrumental in helping me get my first big grant and supported my academic advancement. He had coined the phrase "a culture of compassion" to describe the spirit of volunteerism at our school. In fact, his greatest source of pride as dean occurred when our school was awarded the American Association of Medical Colleges' first-ever Community Service Award. All things considered, we hoped we'd find a receptive ear.

Bernie listened intently, poured over the photos we brought with us, and asked a few questions about the political climate. Finally, it was time for his judgment.

"Sounds great guys. Just stay out of trouble and don't ask me for any money."

For the next two years, Medishare found its way. We knew we wanted to help but we were not sure that we wanted to do. We worked with missionary groups. We work with the Haitian government but we were continually frustrated by lack of partners and opportunities.

In the course of twenty trips, I discovered there were two Haitis—the political Haiti you read about in the newspaper, and the real Haiti that hardly anyone outside the country ever sees. In the media's version of Haiti, the country was in a perpetual state of political violence and crime. In the real Haiti, at the time, political violence was frequently more symbolic than real, a kind of political theater, usually confined to the capital. Crime in the countryside in those days was practically nonexistent. In Haitian culture the worst thing you could possibly be is a thief, a *volé*. People policed themselves. And if anyone should seriously break the rules, there was always the threat of the zombie curse.

But the health situation was dire, especially outside of the capital.

"As bad as it is in Port au Prince, it's worse in the countryside," Miriam had told us on our first visit. "The people there have nothing-no water, no sanitation, no medicine, no electricity, and no roads." After seeing Cite du Soleil, I was skeptical that anything could be worse.

On my fourth trip to Haiti Miriam encouraged me to come out to Pestel and see for myself.

The drive from Port au Prince to the western coastal city of *Au Cayes*, covering one hundred and ten miles on a poorly paved road, took four hours. (*Au Cayes* is the Kreyol name; in French it is *Les Cayes*.) After spending the night in Au Cayes, we embarked in our four-wheel-drive vehicles, equipped with altimeters, inclinometers, and internal/external thermometers, on the fifty-mile, five-hour journey across the mountains that form the spine of Haiti's southern peninsula to the coastal village of Pestel. The following morning, Aussibien, a Haitian boat captain, took us in his sailboat to Caymite, Au Basse, and Z'Etoit.

Each mile we traveled sharpened the contrast between the natural beauty of Haiti and the poverty its people must contend with. The southern peninsula is lush compared to the rest of the country. We saw mountains tumbling into the sea; beaches whose only signs of human presence were abandoned dugout canoes; and forests of palms, vanilla, orchids, and Poinciana. Not far from Port au Prince we noticed small houses scattered through the countryside, with families cooking over open charcoal fires. Women washed their clothes while their children bathed in a low-lying aqueduct built by the side of the road. People traveled on foot, on donkeys, or in impossibly crammed multicolored buses. There was a perfumed scent in the air that mingled with the scent of charcoal, diesel, and cooking oil. "What's that?" I asked our driver.

"*Vetivert,*" he responded, "a perfumed grass that grows in abundance on the southern peninsula. The peasants ship it to France, and it's distilled into perfume." I could make out the large trucks hauling this in front of us, heading for Les Cayes. As we traveled into the interior, the road became rockier and steeper, the houses smaller, more fragile. We passed through Camp Perrin, a small town that looked like it belonged in a western movie, complete with wooden sidewalks and hitching posts in front of its main buildings. We bought some supplies at the general store and then ascended up the mountains.

The altimeters registered three thousand feet. We pulled off by the side of the road halfway between Les Cayes and Pestel for a "deworming clinic." High in the mountains, people live in huts constructed of thatched and woven palm fronds, connected to each other by footpaths. Miriam was right: There was no water, electricity, or sanitation. Yet the people had their families, their traditions, and their little plots of land–their birthright. The government back in Port au Prince could do little to help them, but neither did it oppress them. Mostly, the government seemed invisible way up there. Alongside the crushing poverty, there was pride and hope. Tité called out in Creole to the nearest hut. The mother there sent her four children scurrying towards us and called out to the next hut. Within ten minutes, "teledyol" (Creole for "word of mouth" had produced fifty children.

All the children had the red hair and swollen bellies of malnutrition. According to the routine, they each got a dose of piperazine syrup (we brought gallons), followed by a chunk of bread and then a piece of candy. I was entrusted with this last task. If the candy were unwrapped, there was no problem. If, however, I gave a child candy in a wrapper, he or she stared at me with a look that asked, "What do I do with this?" I had to teach them how to take the wrapper off before they would eat the candy.

We stopped for lunch in the village of Joli Gilbert. Miriam had set up a small malnutrition station there and owned a piece of land on which she hoped to build a clinic one day. From there we could look all the way down the northern slope of the mountain to the village of Pestel below. We unloaded our supplies at the malnutrition center while the woman who worked there prepared a meal for us in her home on the other side of the road. It was the first home in rural Haiti I had been invited into.

The walls were made of wattle and daub, whitewashed inside and out, with blue trim. The roof was thatched palm and the floor hard-packed dirt. The furnishings in the front room (we did not enter the back room, which served as a communal bedroom) were sparse—a homemade table, some homemade ladder-back chairs with rush-matted seats, and a charcoal pot over which she was cooking us a lunch of rice, beans, and chicken. Lunch was interrupted by the sound of singing from the road outside. "Oh, it's a wedding!" exclaimed Miriam, evidently recognizing something about the hymns being chanted by the procession. We left our lunch to wish the bride and groom well—she in her formal bridal dress, he in a tuxedo, both riding mules behind a double line of singing, palm-carrying guests.

After lunch we rapidly descended a rocky road that traversed the slope down to Pestel. We wanted to be settled in by nightfall. Arriving just as market day was winding down in the village square; we inched past throngs of people on foot and on mules heading in the opposite direction.

Pestel had a beautiful natural harbor surrounded by a riot of colorful, ramshackle buildings. The town cistern was broken, so even in this large town there was no water. Electricity came on only sporadically, Miriam explained.

The streets in the main square were still clogged with people, engaged in end-of-the-day buying and selling. The harbor was full of dugout canoes. A small island on the other side of the harbor was rimmed with minuscule houses. Six wooden sailboats, in various stages of construction, lined the waterfront. Four recently completed boats lay at anchor.

We rented a canoe to paddle over to the island and inspect the sailboats. They were totally made by hand—their thick planks ripped from logs with handsaws, the ribs carved with axes, the seams of the sails stitched by hand. The spaces between the planks were caulked with rags; then the boats were filled with saltwater, making the wood swell and the boat watertight. The colors—vivid blues, yellows, and greens—were the same as I had seen on the sailboats used by the boat people seeking refuge in Miami fifteen years earlier.

We spent the next day making "house calls" on remote islands off the coast of Haiti---*Caymite, Au Bas*, and *Z'Etoit*--where most people had never seen a doctor in their entire lives. Everywhere, families kept inviting us into their homes to see their loved ones-people with malaria, tuberculosis, and worms diagnosed without x-rays or laboratory tests. AIDS seemed invisible, very far away, something to worry about on a future trip.

How providential it seemed that, for no logical reason, we appeared at that time to help so many people we met. But how diabolical that so much time had passed before we arrived and how much more time might pass before our return. And Haiti, although poor, was not the poorest spot in the world or the most isolated. There were other places where conditions were probably worse, where there is nothing and no one to alleviate the suffering. At least this place had Miriam and her organization.

The last patient I saw that day was in the most peripheral home in *Z'Etoit,* the furthermost village we visited. The family insisted I see her, claiming she was gravely ill. I entered a small, two-room house with a dirt floor, one door, and no windows. My patient was sitting on the floor in a brown dress, the color of the floor. The dim light made it difficult to see her, except for her eyes and her smile. Although her family referred to her as a child, she was obviously a mature woman. She was retarded, with a small head, and both legs paralyzed. Her family obviously took good care of her. She was clean and well nourished.

Why have they asked me to see her? I thought to myself. She's had this problem from birth. They must think I have magical powers, that I can just lay my hands on her head and restore her to health, that I might be more powerful than a bòkor.

"Nou pa kapab fè plis. Bon kouraj" ("We can't do any better than you. Take heart"), I told her family members, who surrounded me and hoping for a miracle.

As is their custom, everyone thanked us, whether we helped or not. They fed us and sheltered us in their homes. They gathered at the dock to wave goodbye and sang to us as we departed. And I thanked them in return, though I'm not sure they understood why, as we began our long journey back to Miami.

As gratifying as the trip was, it was also troubling. On the one hand, it was a return to the pure joy of being a doctor, unburdened by the bureaucracy and liability and insurance issues that were stultifying my practice in Miami. But I was frustrated by my limited fluency in Creole and by my inability to practice without the bare essentials of medical technology taken for granted at home. And Medishare needed a home of its own, a place that no one else was serving, that no one else wanted.

27
Delva

Project Medishare had been in operation for two years when I first met Delva. He was one three members of the *Komité Zamni Thomonde*–Friends of Thomonde Committee—who came to visit me in my office. All three wore long-sleeve white shirts, red and black ties, and black trousers. Their hometown of Thomonde, located on Haiti' central plateau, northwest of Port au Prince, is more than just a village. It also a "commune," roughly equivalent to a county, that includes four other villages and the surrounding countryside, with approximately 50,000 residents. Historically, in the eyes of the government in Port au Prince, Thomonde did not exist.

Delva was the *Majistrat* (magistrate or mayor) in Thomonde. His two associates were Haitian-Americans living in Miami, although originally from the same area. They had heard that Barth had arranged for Jackson

Memorial Hospital to donate four huge generators to Project Medishare. We had decided to offer them to any Haitian entity that could demonstrate need and promised to maintain them. There is an expression in Creole: Lespwa fé viv, "Hope makes us live." Delva was clearly pinning a lot of his hopes for Thomonde on obtaining one of our generators. He was a short, stocky man who spoke with that perpetual smile that reminded me of Regis. There had been no electricity in Thomonde for more than 20 years, which hindered health and community development. Delva then rattled off a string of statistics documenting just how bad things were in Thomonde and how much good could be accomplished--refrigeration, a hospital, improved education, jobs—if only they had power.

"That's very impressive," I told the committee after Delva finished his presentation, "but it doesn't work like that. It's not within my power to just give you one of these generators. Everyone wants one, and everyone claims they need one. You have to write a proposal. It's competitive. The generators will be awarded according to merit."

The committee members conferred among themselves for a minute.

"No problem," Delva said. "We will have it to you by tomorrow morning."

Delva returned at 8:30 the following morning with a twenty-page plan to bring electricity to Thomonde. He asked if I would review it to be sure it was what I wanted. It was the best proposal had received. Still, I had questions.

"If I give you one of these generators, Delva, how will I know it is actually being used as you have written here?"

"Dr. Fournier, you have my word and an invitation to be my guest in Thomonde whenever you wish. You will stay in my home."

Six months later I received a letter stating that the Thomonde generator had, indeed, arrived, been set up, and was functioning. Delva ended by repeating his invitation to visit Thomonde. I decided to take him up on his offer.

The health statistics Delva provided in his application were appalling: five thousand cases of active tuberculosis. Eighty-five percent of the children malnourished. No health care providers or facilities for 50,000 people. Perhaps this was the "place of our own" Medishare was looking for. In any event, the place--Thomonde, so isolated and remote and the person – Delva, so sincere and determined-intrigued me. How improbable that from the middle of nowhere with no modern means of communication with the outside world, he discovered we had generators to give, found his way to Miami, successfully competed for one, and not only got it back to Haiti but got it back up to the town, which I was told was six hours from Port au Prince on one of the world's worst roads. And then he was polite enough to write me, when he could have just taken the generator, sold it on the black market, and put the cash in his pocket.

Delva met me at the airport as he had promised. We rented a four-wheel drive vehicle; stopped at a gas station for ice, water, and supplies; and headed out for Thomonde. Shortly after leaving Port au Prince, a large green sign marks the point where National Road 3 branches off, threading through the interior of Haiti to Thomonde, Hinche, and points beyond, as if National Route 3 was a real road, perhaps even a highway. Shortly after the sign the pavement ends and the road becomes a dust/dirt/rock/hole/puddle obstacle course that crosses a desert, three mountain ranges, several rivers (some with bridges, some without), and a savannah, finally ending in the city of Cap Haitien.

Haiti is a small country about the size of New Jersey. But it deserves to be a country nonetheless, not only for the uniqueness of its language, history, and culture but also for the fact that it physically takes so long to traverse, making it seem larger than it really is. Delva warned me that his six-hour time estimate from Port au Prince to Thomonde was just that. The trip, if complicated by breakdowns, mud holes, tap-tap turnovers, or washouts, could take twice as long. Recent improvements have cut the time to three and a half hours, but for the last hour and a half it still lives up to its reputation as the worst road in the world.

After *Croix des Bouquets* the road crosses an arid plain carpeted with cacti and thorn acacia trees, then ascends rapidly up the face of *Mòrn Kabri* (Goat Mountain). This is one of the most desolate regions of Haiti, yet there was still a steady stream of people—some on foot, some on horse or mule, and a seemingly endless stream of trucks so top heavy with people and produce that each one seemed destined to topple over at every twist and turn of the road. White limestone dust raised by these trucks coated everything—rocks, vegetation, people—along the way and obscured the view of the road as it hugged the side of the mountain. When we reached the summit, we were greeted with a spectacular view of *Lac Cayman, La Plaine,* Port au Prince, and the mountains of the south beyond. The far side of the mountain turned greener as we descended toward the Val Artibonite.

The way of life, as seen from the road, was correspondingly less harsh: men working rice paddies with sticks to plant and hoes to plow, women with straw hats and hand-made livery riding burros to market. Wide deserted stretches of the road inexplicably transformed into impromptu markets, with thousands of vendors and buyers and piles of rich Haitian produce—eggplant, carrots, onions, and mangoes, freshly butchered goats, and still-living-but-doomed chickens and guinea hens. The road followed the river and the continuing flow of Haitian life in the countryside—women washing clothes and people of all ages, but particularly children, swimming and bathing. Around noon the schools let out and suddenly the road was flooded with children, clustered in color-coded uniforms (each school with its own color) walking hand in hand.

Later, we passed through Mirebalais, a fair-sized town for the area, and stopped for a Haitian cola at a roadside restaurant near the cathedral. Above *Mirebalais* the river valley steepened into a canyon, and the once-tranquil river boiled with cascades and rapids. After we passed the abandoned cement mixers and the dam that created *Lac Peligre* (Danger Lake), the road once again climbed the side of one of the mountains that surround the lake. Since the road here was only rocks, there was no dust, and the view was breathtaking—a huge mountain lake surrounded by peaks on three sides, with the Dominican Republic off in the distance. The lake was dotted with fishermen in dugout canoes. Tiny unpainted wattle and daub houses clung to the hillside between the road and a cliff that tumbled into the lake. Each home had a family outside carrying on their affairs in full view of the neighbors. At the crest of the peak the road left the lakeside and we found ourselves at the small town of *Cange*, home of a health care facility known as *Klinik Bon Sauveur.*

Delva stopped the truck. He wanted me to meet someone. As we entered Delva whispered to me as if we were in church.

"Dr. Paul–he's a very good doctor."

28
Dr. Paul

When Project Medishare was first organized, I contacted several other medical schools to find out who had been working in Haiti. From the many names I learned, Dr. Paul Farmer clearly stood out. He had a combined degree in anthropology and medicine from Harvard and had been working in Haiti for twelve years. He spent six months each year at *Klinik Bon Saveur.* He had written books about his work in Haiti and used the proceeds to support his clinic. His dean (whom I happened to know through a mutual friend) had told me that Dr. Paul was the only living saint he had ever known. His professional life—indeed, even his personal life—reflected total commitment to what he called "a preferential option for the poor,"—a belief that poor people had the same right to health as the rich and shouldn't get second-class care.

Klinik Bon Saveur sat on a promontory overlooking Lac Peligre. Its architecture was half functioning hospital and half gothic monastery.

"Leave it to Harvard to nail down the prime real estate," I joked, to break the ice.

Paul launched into an apology (in the philosophical sense) about the clinic and the people it served. The people in the village we saw as we drove up were all squatters. They had been flooded out of their ancestral homes when the Duvalier government built the dam that created *Lac Peligre*. Built with money from the U.S. Agency for International Aid, the dam was intended to generate hydroelectric power for Port au Prince. Of course, that never happened: No one figured out how to keep the intake valves clear.

"So that's progress in Haiti," deadpanned Paul. "The power never worked and the people lost their land. There is a lot of poverty here in Haiti, but that's the difference between decent poverty and indecent poverty. Land is the Haitian peasant's birthright. For years the United States was afraid Haiti would go communist, so they poured millions to prop up the Duvalier regime. In the process, millions were displaced from their land. No longer able to subsist and support their families, they slipped into the squatter state you saw as you approached."

I made a mental note not to joke with Paul ever again.

I asked him how we might work together. Paul is all about service. He was not interested in our student volunteers. They only slowed him down, and it was a rare student who was culturally competent. Similarly, he was not that interested in training Haitian doctors. He was very cynical about their motivation to work for the poor. He was intrigued, however, about a partnership for Thomonde, which happened to be his biggest problem. Without access to health care, the people there were close enough to Cange to come when desperately ill but not close enough to come for routine care. Thomonde's population dwarfed that of Cange.

Paul's statistics documented the problem. Those estimated five thousand cases of active tuberculosis in Thomonde were only one example.

So Paul said it would please him greatly if some group like Medishare were to adopt Thomonde and work with Delva and the people there to develop a permanent health care system. As he walked us back to our truck after the meeting ended, Paul gave me his gentle admonition not to make a promise and then never come back. It stuck in my mind.

"If you do that, you'll break the people's hearts."

Thomonde was fifteen kilometers, or an hour's ride, after the crest of Cange. As we rounded a ridge I could see that Thomonde lay at the bottom of a huge volcanic caldera, a green oasis amid the grasslands and deforestation of the central plateau. The main village of Thomonde was a pick-up-sticks scattering of streets and cross streets, each lined with traditional Haitian two-room homes—a living room and a communal bedroom. Most were painted bright turquoise with white trim. A large mapou tree decorated with voodoo symbols marked the first fork in the road. Delva's house was of similar design but totally white, with a large tournelle—a large round open space covered by a roof-that served as a village gathering place.

Thomonde was originally settled by the Spanish in 1630. They were probably pushed out by "maroons," runaway slaves in the 1700s. The name Thomonde was derived from the Spanish todo el mundo (all the world). The reason to give this name to a town so isolated escaped me. Somehow, Todo El Mundo changed into Thomonde, roughly transliterated to "Tom's world." It was built on the French village model, with a town square in front of a church at the center of town. Delva took pride in the town square, a small park, and a gazebo that he built with money from the European Union. He introduced me to the village notables and then asked me to address the village via megaphone from the gazebo. I met the vice-mayors and the schoolteachers, and Bernardeau, a local success story who had emigrated to Boston years earlier and sold used cars. Now he was wealthy by Thomonde's standards and returned to Thomonde every winter to avoid Boston's chill. A party erupted with dancing and rum and clapping. Project Medishare, in the person of Dr. Fournier, had come to Thomonde.

Delva gave up his bed and home and moved in with a neighbor for the night. I marveled at the workmanship of the shutters and the doors of Delva's house. When the kerosene in the lamp burned out, I was left in the darkness with my thoughts. Voodoo drums pounded in the distance. Their rhythm and intensity helped me focus. Here was a place no one else wanted but a place that wanted us, a place where Project Medishare could make a difference.

Before we left Thomonde to return to Port au Prince, Delva took me to make a house call on his parents. They lived in a small house on the edge of town, with a surprisingly large plot of land, neatly demarcated by cactus hedge rows. His father had suffered a stroke in the recent past, and his mother had some pain in her left shoulder that caused Delva some concern.

Before examining them, Delva introduced me and pulled over a hand-made ladder-back chair for me to sit on. His mother had been cooking soup for her husband over a charcoal fire outside. She was short and, like Delva, always smiling. Instead of the usual head wrap, she wore a cheery blue broad-rimmed bonnet. She beamed with pride as I told them the story of the generator and Delva's first trip to Miami. There wasn't much I could do for his father. The stroke had crippled his right side and made it extremely difficult for him to speak. The smell of urine permeated his bedclothes. I suggested he take an aspirin a day and that the family try to get him out of bed as much as possible. His mother had a simple case of tendonitis. I gave her an anti-inflammatory medicine that I had in my suitcase. In half an hour her pain was gone--Medishare's first success in Thomonde.

29
Tom's World

Six weeks later I was back.

... *"Ti Poul*, Delva! *Ti Poul!"* cried Susan S. from the passenger side of our rented truck. She clutched the dashboard as if it were a brake lever. "Pa gen pwoblem," chuckled Delva as he swerved the truck to avoid the latest mother hen and chicks to dare cross our path as we bounded and crunched our way from Pignon to Thomonde. The swerve lifted us out of the rut that traffic had worn in the dirt road. Although Delva was accommodating to Susan's desire not to kill any chickens, he was not going to slow down. We had to get to Thomonde. There would be lots of patients waiting.

"Ti Poul-yo," I corrected Susan's Creole. "There is more than one chicken." It had become a running joke now: Susan's "I brake for animals" vigilance balanced between Delva's determination to complete the

four-hour road trip from Thomonde to Pignon to Thomonde by 10:00 a.m. Every time we bounced on a boulder the students in the truck bay would scream "Yahoo!" Children watched us cautiously from behind their cactus hedge rows or ran laughing after us yelling, "Gadé, blan! Gadé blan!" (Look at the strangers!)

Seeing *"blan yo"* in this part of Haiti, deep in the interior, close to the Dominican border, eight miles from anywhere, was certainly an event. I had kept my promise to Delva to come back with a team of medical students to a health fair in Thomonde. By screening for common, preventable, treatable problems, such as worms and malnutrition, we could start the process of returning health to Thomonde. Project Medishare was not an official part of the University of Miami's curriculum. But word was passing from student to student that there was a real opportunity to learn in Haiti. As a consequence, more and more students were giving up their spring, summer, and winter breaks and volunteering for Medishare. On this trip I had 12 second-year medical students, long on book knowledge but short on experience. I was the only real doctor. But that was the wonderful thing about the health fair method: One doctor aided by a dozen students could see a lot of patients.

Delva showed me the Uzi he kept under his seat. As mayor of Thomonde he wanted us to know that he personally guaranteed our safety while visiting Thomonde. The students were impressed with the Uzi, particularly since the Miami Herald had written another series of articles about gang violence and police ineffectiveness in Port au Prince just before our trip. Delva was more concerned about reports that there were barricades blocking the road around Hinche. The report turned out to be nothing more than rumor. Neither barricades nor gangs ever materialized. I wasn't worried.

We pulled off the road and into the field that surrounded the newly finished magistrate's office. Hundreds of people who had gathered outside cheered our arrival, at exactly 10:00 a.m. The day before we had seen about two hundred children—plotted their heights and weights, identified those who were malnourished, and treated the ones with worms and impetigo. We had promised the gramoun (the adults) that we would see them today, but first we had to transport the sickest children to the hospital in Pignon, about two hours away. Some of the students stayed behind to give health education classes on malnutrition, oral rehydration, family planning, and HIV prevention.

"N'ap kòmanse nan senk minet. Mesi pou pasyans ou!" ("We'll start in five minutes. Thanks for your patience!"), I announced as I pushed through the crowd and past the iron gate entrance to our makeshift clinic. "How'd the classes go?" I asked the students gathered in the central foyer. "Great! You could tell by the questions the patients asked that they were really getting it. Jean-Gason and Jean-Peter [two boys from the local school who were fluent in English and had volunteered to translate] did a super job!" volunteered Susan A.

"But Dr. F. We've got a problem."

"What's that?"

"All those people want to be seen," he said. "We counted nearly six hundred."

"Well, I guess we'd better see them. We've got twelve students, so that means two students in each exam room, plus two to guard the gate and regulate patient flow, and two to man the dispensary. Organize yourselves, and let's get started."

The crowd was already pressing against the iron gate, but the people backed adjust enough for me to exit and announce, *"Gramoun premyé!"* (Old folks first!). In Haitian culture old people are revered. Gramoun, which means "old person," also means "wise person." Adhering to this tradition, we decided to see the oldest patients first. The sea of people in front of the gate parted as four men carried in the oldest citizen of Thomonde on a palette and helped her into an easy chair.

"Bonjour, Dokté," she said as she was carried by me. *"Bonjou, Mami,"* I responded. "Susan, Felix—would you please take this first patient? Use Jean Peter to help you."

Remarkably, in ten minutes the clinic was in high gear. The students performed limited histories and physical examinations, while I rotated from room to room, identifying the problems and how we'd treat them. Then the patients would go to the "dispensary" (a table set up in the central foyer with the essential medicines we had brought from Miami) to pick up their medicine. The only problem was that there was only one gate out, and everyone was trying to get in.

"Dr. F., This first patient says she's 115 years old. Could that be right?"

"It's probably pretty close, since her daughter who's with her tells me she's 84."

"What do you want us to do for her?"

"Find out why she can't walk. Do a complete exam. Don't worry, take your time."

After an hour it was clear that the patients had four general types of problems—Bouton, gratél and other skin conditions, high blood pressure, heart problems, fevers, masses, hernias. Though the makeshift clinic was running pretty smoothly, we had a major problem: how to get the patients we had already seen out without letting the increasingly anxious crowd in.

"We've finished our exam and don't find anything terribly wrong," said Susan A. "She's just a little unsteady on her feet," referring to the 115-year-old woman. I stopped my running from room to room when it hit me.

"That's the oldest person I've ever met and probably ever will."

I went over to talk to her—a sweet woman who looked remarkably like her daughter. She would like to walk but was afraid of falling, she said. We had brought a walker from Miami which we gave her. Five minutes later, the 115-year-old woman who was carried in walked out under her own power. The crowd roared its approval.

This seeming miracle, though, only increased each person's desire to be seen, so the crowd pushed even harder to get through the gate. *"Pa pouse, Pa pouse!"* I called out ("Don't push!") David and Tom were leaning all of their weight against the gate to keep it shut. Finally, the hinges gave way. The five hundred citizens of Thomonde still waiting to be seen poured through the gate and down the two corridors of the magistrate's office.

"All of you, stop seeing patients!" I screamed as I withdrew to the central foyer. "Gather up your things! We need to get out of here!"

In five minutes, as the last of the patients streamed in, the students and I were able to march out, single file, carrying our precious medicines in duffel bags. I announced in Creole that people needed to leave the magistrate's office immediately or we would never return to Thomonde again.

It seemed like I was the only one who took the situation seriously. The patients were laughing and the students were smiling, amazed by the spectacle of it all, as we retreated towards the truck. A circus atmosphere prevailed. Delva, who had been working on making us lunch, came running over from his house, looking worried. *"Kisa k'ap rivé?"* (What's going on?), he asked me as he caught his breath.

"Yon ti revolusyon, se tou" (Just a little revolution, that's all), I responded. Delva's voice obviously carried more authority than mine. *"Sòti kounye-a!"* (Get out now!), he barked, and in minutes his office was empty again. He told the patients we were going to take a lunch break and reorganize, that we'd return and would attempt to see everyone, once we had established a reasonable plan.

Delva whisked us away in the truck to a secret place—a relative's house—where we huddled to see how we could solve the patient flow problem. We returned to Delva's office by 3:00. We had the patients form four lines—one for skin problems, one for heart/blood pressure, one for fevers, and one for masses and hernias. These groupings were important. Although it's true that few people died of skin problems, the misery they caused was extreme and they were easy to treat, which would build confidence among our patients in Western medicine. The fever line was critical. With a few simple questions we could sort out patients with malaria, which we could treat on the spot, from those with suspected tuberculosis, whom we'd have to send "en masse" to Dr. Paul in Cange. The "hernia line" might seem trivial, but with the only surgeon in the region two hours away in Pignon, I knew that we'd find a lot that had never been repaired. In Thomonde, a hernia could keep you from working, and if you couldn't work, you couldn't feed your family. Each student team was assigned to a single line, with each line forming outside a single room. We were back in business again, each line moving at a noticeable pace, and no pushing, or pressing.

30
Exposition Santé

That was Project Medishare's first health fair in Thomonde. We've subsequently returned, about three times per year, with an ever-growing cadre of committed students. The early health fairs were pretty chaotic events. Michel and I were the most consistent trip leaders. In a community that had received health care only episodically from missionaries, we had to break through an unspoken communal mind-set in which every patient pushed to be seen, shared a litany of complaints, and hoped to walk away with some magic pill, any pill. It didn't matter whether it would really help them or not.

In the beginning, malnutrition was rampant in Thomonde. It was easy to screen for: Simply line up all the children with red hair. Hair is, in essence, pure protein. The first signs of protein deficiency show in hair. The hair of malnourished children in Haiti changes from curly, thick, and black to thin, sparse, and red. Human beings are 95 percent water. One of the many miraculous things that protein does is to keep water in our cells and circulatory system, rather than us dissolving into an amorphous puddle. As protein deficiency progresses, therefore, a child's belly and feet swell with fluid. Malnutrition is further complicated by worms. When we first went to Thomonde, we just assumed each child had worms. Therefore, each health fair in the early days always had a de-worming line. The red hair and swollen bellies of malnutrition were not just clinical signs of the disease; they were signs for all to see that these children were somehow marked for misfortune and probably premature death.

One family was particularly poignant—two devoted parents and five daughters, all under the age of five, all slowly starving to death. I explained to my students how the mother had breast-fed each child but had to stop prematurely to return to her work selling produce in the market. With this many children, none could be adequately nourished. As I was telling the mother what kinds of foods she should be giving her children, she burst into tears. Her children were marked by a particularly unusual sign of malnutrition: Their hair turned not red but blonde!, and she blamed herself. Worse, there was nothing she could do about it, as the family was too poor even to raise chickens, let alone goats or a pig. I was ashamed of my insensitivity. Before I left them, I touched her hand and whispered *"kenbe,"* a Creole expression that means "hang in there."

Riding back to Port au Prince, one of the students, Stephanie, volunteered that her husband worked for a company, Rexall-Sundown, which made vitamins and protein supplements. She would write a letter to the president of the company, requesting a donation. Stephanie's letter resulted in a donation of fourteen palettes (approximately two tons) of multivitamins and protein supplements. With the help of a Peace Corps volunteer, we started feeding and prenatal care programs. Shortly thereafter, the kids in Thomonde started having black hair again.

Over time our health fairs became more organized. We started going out to the remote corners of the commune: to villages of *Tierre Muscadet, Savannette,* and *Bas Touribe,* one of the most isolated places on the planet. Totally cut off from everything but Thomonde and Cange, not even within range of the nearest radio station, it's surprising the Bas Touribois have not evolved their own language. With no electricity or cars, the people live in a timeless, traditional way. Most *Bas Touribois* rarely travel more than ten kilometers from the place of their birth during their entire lifetime. We began doing our health fairs in the church in *Bas Touribe,* a cool shady place, with a good breeze when its doors are open. The priest let us use his vestibule–a small room off the altar–for Pap smear screening.

Pap smears had never been done in this part of Haiti–a Project Medishare first. We found a lot of positives, but imagine the difficulty of explaining the need for and the process of such a procedure to people in such remote place. So we started with a class in Creole that began with the basics: What is a cell? What is cancer? Does anyone know someone who died of cancer? Hundreds of women lined up and patiently waited all day for their turn to climb up on the makeshift examining table and submit to the examination. Pap smear screenings continue today.

While the students set up for the screening, I circulated in the crowd, explaining that we're not there to treat every ache and pain but to screen for problems that might kill them. I also scan the throngs for the obviously ill who need to receive individual attention. They're easy to identify with their wasted frames and gaunt, frightened stares. The patients I can visually identify as having AIDS or tuberculosis invariably are standing off by themselves, shunned by the crowds. In Haiti, failing health can only be explained by a curse. Both the victims and their neighbors understand that.

The health fairs proved to be great for screening and prevention. They were also a clever way to engage and organize our enthusiastic but inexperienced medical students. Since Medishare had first come to

Thomonde, we had brought the commune from no health care to episodic care, with screening and patient education. Episodic care was certainly better than no care at all, but the visiting American doctors and students were never going to break through the stigma and shame of AIDS, tuberculosis, and malnutrition. We needed a permanent presence. And it would have to be Haitian.

31
Benediction

Driving on Haitian roads demands the complete attention of all of one's senses. So the questions of my students were somewhat of a distraction as I drove to the town of *Croix des Bouquets,* in early 2001. Potholes, pedestrians, and poliz stasyone (speed bumps) lurked ahead, while in the opposite direction "tap-taps" of every color and dimension rushed toward us bumping, jerking, and narrowly missing us at every turn. On the other hand, I'd never felt more alive. Nothing seemed impossible.

We were driving to *Croix des Bouquets* to read tuberculin tests at an orphanage. In seven years, Project Medishare had grown from a small volunteer organization to a charity sponsoring major programs in community health in Thomonde and in training Haitian doctors to be family physicians in *Cap Haitien* and *Pignon.* At the same time, we maintained an ongoing commitment to provide health care services to a cluster of orphanages near Port au Prince. Support for our charity had grown steadily. Initially funded predominantly by contributions from Barth and to a lesser extent by me, we were becoming more and more successful with our art auctions and with grants and donations from the community. Furthermore, we impressed on our students the need to raise funds—at least what was required to pay their own way.

A cohesive plan was starting to evolve. Michel and I wrote a grant to establish a family medicine training program in Haiti. The billionaire George Soros funded it. The first class of Haitian residents was at work at *Cap Haitien* and *Pignon*. Meanwhile more than one hundred medical students had volunteered for Project Medishare in Thomonde. Between the orphanages, the residency program, and Thomonde, we were poised to make a difference. There was no denying that Haitians were still dying in boats trying to get to Florida, that AIDS was still creating orphans, that the news out of Port au Prince was perpetually bad, and that the "powers that be" at our medical school still didn't get what Medishare was all about. We were making a difference. The finally completed guesthouse in Thomonde exceeded everyone's expectations, not just in terms of comfort but also in expanding our capacity to work in the village of Thomonde and its surrounding communities. Students from other medical schools, coming to Miami for fourth-year experiences called externships from as far away as Saskatchewan, heard about our Haiti experiences and signed on.

"What about the elections?" came a voice from the back of the van.

"They're going to happen," I answered.

The Miami press was all wrapped up in the impending legislative and municipal elections. Was Aristide stalling, so that one combined presidential and legislative election would sweep Lavalas into power at all levels?

"None of our business," I told the students. "Too much of Haitian politics starts and ends in Washington." What this election flap is all about is whether there will be a 'globalization' of the Haitian economy.

Aristide was elected by promising jobs for the poor and taxes for the rich. After the coup and his expulsion, accommodation with globalization was the price he had to promise in exchange for a United Nations intervention to return him to power. The Haitian peasants couldn't care less about the World Bank or globalization of their economy. Furthermore, the bloom was off the rose of globalization. It was not working the miracles it promised, and its cost is being carried on the backs of the people.

Meanwhile, as Paul Farmer had explained to me, fifty years of American foreign policy toward Haiti had been shaped by the fear that Haiti would go communist. Cuba had gone communist, and according to theory, Haiti, even poorer, was certain to follow. But anyone with a modicum of knowledge of Haitian history knew Haiti would never go communist. To Haitian peasants the land was their birthright, the gift of their ancestors' revolution. They would never give it up. So for that misreading of history we supported Duvalier and the generals.

"If you want to help Haiti," I said, "ignore the politics and focus one on one on our humanitarian mission. Given enough time without outside influence, the Haitians will fix their own politics. It won't be easy, but it's the only way."

"I don't understand this birthright thing, Dr. Fournier," came a challenging voice from the back of the truck. "And this liberation theology preached by President Aristide. It sure does sound a lot like socialism."

"In 1815, Haiti's leaders tried to revive the plantation economy," I replied. "They enacted 'land reforms' that would have tied the former slaves back to the sugar fields and a state of serfdom. The peasants voted with their feet. They took off into the mountains, carved up the land among themselves, and passed it on from generation to generation. In effect, they traded a subsistence existence for their freedom. Aristide and his liberation theology have to be seen in the context of two hundred years of struggle between the poor and the elite for what they both consider their birthright. But trust me–the Haitian peasants will never give up their land. The problem is, with the average family having five kids, the birthright gets smaller and smaller and subsistence gets harder and harder."

Silence descended on the van as the students pondered my diatribe. It was great to see how much they learned in only a week, not just about medicine but also about Haiti, the world, and themselves. Past the wattle and daub huts, the piles of watermelons, the hand-woven baskets, and the continuous stream of life on the National Road, we raced from the north toward *Croix des Bouquets*. As we passed the remains of Ibo Beach, I pointed out where sexually active tourists had most likely introduced HIV to Haiti, then the salt flats where the bodies of Duvalier's victims were left for the crabs to scavenge, and the trash dumps where children still forage for scraps to this day.

Thank you, Haiti, I thought that day, I had the zombie curse of a comfortable life in the United States. For all my good intentions, I was in a kind of spiritual coma. Previlus, Theophile, Marie—I'm trying. Regis—I've not forgotten. Hopefully, we will make a difference.

The Green Family Foundation (no relation to Barth Green) funded Medishare's proposal for a community health project in Thomonde. In partnership with Paul Farmer, we planned to renovate the dispensary and hire Haitian doctors and nurses to bring full-time health care to Thomonde. We also planned to hire a small army of community health workers. Paul would train them in outreach and direct observed therapy, a simple but effective way to make sure sick patients get their medicines. Delva was defeated in his bid for reelection as magistrate so he was available to join our effort. It turned out that in his youth Delva had studied public health and had trained as a tuberculosis control workers. So he would lead our team.

Relations between Medishare and the U of M medical school grew strained. The provost, the general counsel, and the associate dean for education feared the possible liability accrued by students volunteering in Haiti and their perception of the danger our students might face while working in Haiti. These concerns were fueled by a continuing string of sensationalist articles about the political instability in Haiti in the Miami Herald. It seemed that negative articles always appeared in our local newspaper one or two weeks before each trip's departure. On our side, we have Barth, probably the most successful fundraiser the University of Miami had ever seen. We had the example set by Paul Farmer and his relationship to Harvard and our students, who were doing important work on tuberculosis among orphans, sickle-cell anemia, and women's health.

The dean was noncommittal for several months. Who could blame him with the challenges facing the medical center? A grant from the Green Family Foundation tipped the balance in our favor–$250,000 per year for three years to improve the health of Thomonde and a parallel grant to the department of pediatrics to start an international pediatric infectious diseases program. A condition of the award was that the issues between Medishare and the school had to be resolved.

The grant did more than give Medishare leverage at the school. It gave Medishare a permanent health presence in Thomonde, allowing us to break through the limits of what we could accomplish with only episodic visits. The key was not so much the renovated clinic or the Haitian doctors or nurses who would be there full time (although these were all critical advances) but the thirty six community health workers, handpicked by Delva.

He chose them from every corner of the commune–men, women, young and old, former farmers, market women, teachers, and students. The grant provided them with mules and motorcycles that enabled them to visit every household of every district–Thomonde, *Boucan Carrè Savanette, Tierre Muscadet,* and *Bas Touribe.* Trained to a remarkable degree of medical sophistication by Paul, they could identify the ill, bring them to the dispensary for diagnosis and treatment, educate them as peers, and ensure that they would take their medicines. It was health care by the people, of the people, for the people. We paid each worker about

$100 per month, about five times the amount they could earn by farming. With Delva leading them and Paul inspiring them, they took their work with utmost seriousness.

Delva arranged for the Catholic bishop to come down from *Hinche* to bless our guesthouse and clinic. Actually, the guesthouse today is no longer just our guesthouse; it serves as the health care headquarters for our community health workers. It's now the most substantial home in Thomonde, surpassing that of the funeral director. Everything in Haiti has meaning, and the symbolism of this proprietal comeuppance was not lost on the *Thomondois* or, for that matter, on me. Death is a growth industry in rural Haiti, and in practically every town, the largest and most prosperous-looking home always belongs to the funeral director. This is no longer the case in Thomonde. Health now has the upper hand.

The house blessing ceremony included a visit by Paul and his staff from Cange. The ceremony was scheduled for 4:00 in the afternoon, and we spent the day prior to the inauguration giving health care to the citizens of Thomonde. Barth came—his third trip to Haiti with Medishare—and differentiated from neurosurgeon to primary care physician. After conceptualizing Project Medishare and financing and participating in the first trip, he had pretty much turned the project over to me. This was certainly understandable. In addition to running the neurosurgery department, he had launched a campaign to find a cure for paralysis. Now, however, seven years into the project, perhaps because his own children were now volunteering in Medishare, Barth was once again engaged. We had thirty medical students with us. They had worked hard all day, but filled in the back rows of the tournelle during the inauguration, surreptitiously sipping beer and marveling at the event.

Paul arrived early and really hit it off with Barth and the students. He and Barth talked about building a day hospital on the property next to the guesthouse. The bishop said a high mass in French. Afterwards, Barth, Paul, and I were asked to speak. Paul worked the crowd with a rousing speech in Creole, celebrating with the *Thomondois* their participation in living a healthy life.

After mass the bishop passed through the house and blessed it with holy water. The Thomonde brass band, usually relegated only to funerals, played several celebratory songs, including the Haitian and American national anthems. Medical students and the citizens of Thomonde intermingled, drinking beer, and home-brewed clairin, a potent homemade rum. The generator hummed, providing light and music well into the evening. Even Paul let his guard down, socializing with the students and sipping enough beer to start telling jokes and poses for pictures. The Peace Corps volunteers fueled the celebration with a homemade rum punch.

I slipped away to a quiet corner of our property to play the "rock game" with some of Thomonde's children. I always play the rock game with the children. They count on this and sit patiently, twenty to thirty at a time, every evening I spend in Thomonde.

The game is simple. First, I search the ground for a small, shiny rock. Then I line up the children in a row, sitting on their haunches. I place the rock in a hand behind my back and then offer them my two closed fists to choose which one contains the hidden rock. If they choose the hand with the rock, they win. If they choose the empty hand, they lose. I go down the line, and each child gets to choose. Each child gets lots of advice from the others when it is their turn, and each choice right or wrong, is greeted with peals of laughter. "Ou genyen" ("you win"), "*Ou genyen . . . Ou pedi. . .*" ("You lose"), down the line I go. I pass through the line several times, so that each child wins at least once, and then turn the game over to them. That night the rock game went for hours. Haiti, land of contrasts. For all the misery that surrounds them, these children found joy in guessing which hand holds a small rock. Not just a little joy, mind you, but unabashed, unrestrained joy–more joy than could possibly be produced by a million video games. As much as I keep trying to give to Haiti, Haiti–particularly its children keeps giving even more to me. When I awoke the next morning the children were there again, ready to begin at first light. I passed the rock to a young girl who seemed precocious, and I took her place in line, pretending to be a kid again, but this time I felt like a Haitian kid. I won each time.

32
War and Floods

The year 2004 was supposed to be a festival year in Haiti, bicentennial celebration marking two hundred years since its independence from France. The year didn't turn out that way, however. The U.S. media presented the growing rebellion against Aristide in a favorable light and painted the Haitian government as incompetent at best, corrupt, and evil at worst. Aristide, for his part, seemed to be sleepwalking through the crisis. I wondered how many of his nine political lives he had left. Perhaps someone put a zombie curse on him, I thought. Certainly he had made mistakes during his administration. I had become disillusioned with his political party, *Lavalas,* after Delva lost the Thomonde mayoral election. I had no sympathy for the rebels, however. They were clearly mercenaries with a sordid past. Worse, the theatrical violence I had noticed early on as an integral part of the Haitian political landscape was no longer just for show. Lives were being lost.

Inexorably the rebels marched from the north and the central plateau toward Port au Prince. Resistance evaporated in the face of their advance, almost as if the whole rebellion were orchestrated on both sides. When Cap Haitien fell under rebel control, services at our family practice clinic were disrupted for three days. In the Central Plateau our ambulance was "borrowed" by rebel troops three times. Each time, thanks to the consummate negotiating skills of Delva, it was located and returned to Thomonde.

I was shocked to see a picture in the Miami Herald of rebels escorting Red Cross troops through *Gönaives*. The article talked of the "humanitarian crisis" developing in the north as a result of the roads being cut by the rebels and the inability of the Red Cross to deliver emergency food relief. The rebels had let them through in exchange, it seems, for a major photo opportunity. I drafted a protest e-mail to the Red Cross and received a polite letter back, explaining how they could not be effective if they didn't remain neutral. Meanwhile, my Haitian-American friends were advising me to give it up.

"The handwriting is on the wall, Art. The Haitian elite, the U.S. Embassy, and the media are all over Aristide. Remember, after he is gone, you still want to be able to function in the country," one told me.

We were forced to cancel our spring volunteer trip. Communication with Thomonde was sporadic. Marie was marooned in Port au Prince, our e-mail was down, and Delva could only occasionally get to the capital to send us phone messages. Fortunately, our Haitian infrastructure held together. The hospital in *Cange* never shut down. The Thomondois protected our guesthouse and clinic from looting and vandalism. Medical service interruptions were minimal. Through it all, our community health workers slogged it out, assuring that the mundane miracle of direct observed therapy continued.

Eventually, a small contingent of U.S. marines landed. A few days later the United States and France declared they had no confidence in

Aristide and, in the middle of the night, escorted him out of the country. He later claimed he was "kidnapped" by U.S. forces. The bizarre history of the relationship between Haiti and the United States had taken a new turn. When a caretaker Haitian-American prime minister was flown in from Boca Raton, Florida, he hailed the rebels as "freedom fighters."

After four months of headlines about Haiti, the media turned their attention to the presidential campaign and the conflict in Iraq. On the ground in Haiti, things in Port au Prince were as bad or worse than when Medishare first came ten years earlier. There was no electricity. There were huge piles of uncollected garbage. There was political violence. The government was bankrupt. The U.N. peacekeeping forces seemed reluctant to intervene in the simmering feud between polarized political factions. Political turmoil in the winter and spring was followed by natural disasters during the rainy season. In May 2005 flooding killed hundreds in the towns of *Jimani* and *Fonds Verrettes.* In September, floods spurned by tropical storm Jeanne killed thousands and left hundreds of thousands of people homeless in the region around the city of Gonaïves.

The international peacekeeping force and international relief agencies seemed totally unprepared. The United States pledged a paltry $50,000 for humanitarian relief, then increased its pledge to $2 million after it was shamed by more substantive contributions by Venezuela and Cuba. People who had gone without food and water for days were scattered from food distribution centers by rifle shots and tear gas. Marie, Delva, our doctors in Thomonde, and our partners in Cange packed truckloads of medicines and drove them into the disaster area, donating them to the agencies–Care and UNICEF–responsible for recovery.

"It was worse than you could possibly imagine," Marie told me. "The stench of death was everywhere. But almost as bad–depressing, really– was how disorganized the international relief effort was. No one knew what the others were doing; no one took charge. Women and children were walking around in a state of shock."

There are those who believe that events such as the floods of

Gonaïves are proof that Haiti is, indeed, cursed. There is a legend in Haiti that Toussaint L'Overture made a pact with the devil to drive out the French and that all of Haiti's woes spring from that Mephistophelian source. From a theological perspective, the "Haiti is cursed" theory should not be dismissed without careful deliberation. The recurrent flash flooding in Haiti is the result of deforestation of the country. Many Haitians believe that *Lwa,* the Voodoo spirits, live in the trees, particularly mapou and mahogany. Being totally dependent on charcoal for fuel, the Haitian peasants are forced to choose between survival and the wrath of the gods.

But the secret of the zombie curse is that Haiti's curses are not supernatural in origin but rather the consequences of the actions of men. I recalled my conversation with the founder of the Haiti Baptist Mission concerning the mudslides caused by tropical storm Gordon ten years before. Since then a decade had passed and nothing had been done to address the root causes of this kind of disaster. Certainly the cutting of trees for charcoal in the most densely populated country in the Western Hemisphere established conditions that in a major storm like Jeanne could sweep away all in its path. But here, once again, blaming the victim makes it easy for us to walk away. It's the peasants' fault for cutting down the trees, we assume. The real cause of the death and despair of the floods is the same as the AIDS epidemic–poverty and its consequences. Poverty drove the Haitian peasants to try to terrace and till every inch of marginal farmland. Poverty continues to drive them to use the cheapest fuel possible–charcoal, knowing they are killing their country in the process.

Ironically, one area where things have improved, albeit slightly, is the AIDS epidemic. Countrywide, the prevalence of HIV had actually fallen a bit, a blessing that's probably attributable to a falloff in exploitative sexual tourism, new programs in public education, and the superhuman efforts of Paul Farmer, and others engaged in the AIDS education and prevention. Wisely, the people at the U.S. Agency for International

Development realize that the war against AIDS can't be fought in a vacuum. They've designed a countrywide multifaceted program that is creating a general health care infrastructure with the capacity for AIDS care, rather than trying to treat only AIDS. Programs in prevention and nutrition as well as AIDS care and treatment are being implemented.

Project Medishare's family medicine training program is playing a role in this effort. The program provides services to patients in the city of Cap Haitien. We are also training the next generation of Haitian doctors to be competent in all aspects of AIDS care. In 2004, over 1,000 patients with AIDS joined the 15,000 patients already receiving comprehensive health care services from our residents and faculty in Cap Haitien.

In Thomonde, remarkable health progress has been made, despite Haiti's precarious political situation. Paul Farmer received a large grant from the Global Fund to Fight AIDS, Tuberculosis, and Malaria, which has made medicines available to all and allowed us to expand our team of health care workers. With treatment and a simple but effective delivery system (our community health workers), the stigma of AIDS and tuberculosis is dissolving in Thomonde. Over four hundred patients have been enrolled in our direct observed therapy program. To date, not one has died. There are two secrets to our success in Thomonde. First, we've trained Thomondois to be peer educators, counselors, and therapists. This has enabled patients to care for themselves, and take an active role in their own health, with the health care workers serving as a safety net if things don't go according to plan.

My colleagues in Miami think I'm joking when I tell them we now have a better and fairer health care system for the poor in Thomonde than we do in Miami, but I'm serious. How ironic that Thomonde—one of the poorest regions of the poorest country in the hemisphere—has a more effective model of care than most of the United States. In Kreyol there is no verb equivalent to the French avoir, "to have." The closest equivalent is ginyen, meaning to gain or earn. So in Thomonde the people take nothing for granted: One doesn't "have" good health, one earns it. A trip to Thomonde will quickly shatter stereotypes about the poor—that the poor are lazy or dumb or lack family values. The Thomondois as a group are industrious and eager for knowledge about their health. Their entire lives are family centered—materially, in the sense that life evolves around the inherited family plot of land-but also spiritually—children, old folks, and ancestors are all revered. They're also community centered. There's not only a knowledge of and concern for all of one's neighbors but also a communal way of getting things done, whether it's building a house or clearing a field. These are traditions that started in the days of slavery. In this milieu it has been much easier to build a health care system than one might think.

Medishare also supports education and nutrition programs and, most importantly, has created meaningful jobs, perhaps the most effective way to fight the infectious diseases that afflict the poor. We have helped create a rural middle class in the health care sector. Our community health care workers cost us about $100 per month—a pittance by U.S. standards, but a decent salary in a country with an average per capita income of $200 per year. These funds have percolated throughout the commune, contributing to the well being and elevating the standard of living and quality of life.

When Medishare celebrated its tenth anniversary in 2005, it far exceeded my original expectations when I first joined. Every day, starting at 6:00 a.m., our cooks brew several pots of Haitian coffee, scramble eggs, and cook Haitian spaghetti to send off our fifty community health workers on their daily rounds. The workers pack their coolers with ice, so their vaccines won't spoil, and stuff their satchels with Direct Observed Therapy forms and precious medicines. By 7:00 a.m. they set off—some on foot, some by horse, and some by motorcycle—to the farthest reaches of the commune, full of zeal and enthusiasm for their work and a loving concern for their patients that I rarely see anymore in America.

In addition to treating AIDS and tuberculosis, our workers have launched an immunization campaign. In 2002, Thomonde had the worst immunization rates in Haiti. Now, 98 percent of the children have been immunized. If school children show signs of malnutrition, they'll receive a nutritious meal called Akamil at school, in exchange for their parents keeping them enrolled. Pregnant women and patients on DOT also get *Akamil,* flavored with cinnamon and vanilla. The dispensary opens at 9:00. On the average day, two hundred patients pass through its doors.

Meanwhile, before dawn, while the *Lycee* students up in *Cap Haitien* are pacing and reciting their devwa ("homework"), our residents are reviewing their admissions from the night before in anticipation of attending rounds. Patients line up each day at the family practice center for immunization and family planning. The program is now sustained through funding from the U.S. Agency for International Development. Haiti's ministry of health is encouraging us to expand training of family doctors, and we're hoping to open a second program based in Thomonde as soon as we've completed construction of a new hospital and clinic. Blessed with knowledgeable and enthusiastic Haitian partners, we are making a difference.

When University of Miami president Donna Shalala visited Haiti in 2004, the issues between Medishare and the University of Miami vanished. The dean agreed to send a team of eye doctors and students to give eye care to the people of *Cange* and *Thomonde* on a regular basis. Shalala helped us connect with some major international donors. More than a hundred first-year medical students— two-thirds of the class–have signed up to volunteer for Project Medishare. They are busily planning, along with our fifty second-year students, this year's health fairs. Over the years more than five hundred medical students, doctors, and nurses have contributed to Haiti's health under Medishare's umbrella. Other medical schools-notably, George Washington, Emory, and Morehouse – are partnering with us to expand services in the communities around Thomonde.

Our collaboration with Paul Farmer's Partners in Health has allowed us to expand our community health workers and created an environment in which the Haitian doctors and nurses have the backup and support they need. In turn, Paul has hired one of the graduates of our family medicine training program to work in Cange.

"Send me more," he says, when I ask him how our doctor is doing. "He can do it all."

To date, we've graduated thirty five doctors from our residency program in Haiti. All but two are now working as family doctors in the countryside. Medishare will produce at least five Haitian family doctors per year and will hopefully increase that number to ten in the near future.

Medishare owes a lot to Paul Farmer. The example he sets in terms of sacrifice, dedication, cultural competency, and solidarity with the people, plus his commitment to health as an issue of social justice and his unwillingness to accept a double standard of care for poor people, is remarkable. In his writings, Paul eloquently makes the point that when effective treatment exists with unequal access to care there is an injustice. Through our health fairs, patient education programs, immunization campaigns, and training program, Medishare has extended Paul's concept to include not just treatment but also screening, prevention, and primary care. We steadfastly believe that, through education, the torch must be passed to Haitian providers.

Over our first ten years, Medishare volunteers have made more than a hundred trips to Haiti. We have experienced our share of scorching heat, torrential rains, political turmoil, flat tires, and mud holes. We've also had total strangers help us change those tires, pull us out of those mud holes, and shelter us from the tribulations that are part of daily life in one of the poorest countries in the world. In the early days, I frequently traveled alone. Now, I never lack for friends and companions. Invariably, the Haitian people have given much to me--lessons of courage, patience, ingenuity, and mysticism—and countless opportunities to make a difference. Little did I know than that the Haitian values I had absorbed were soon to be put to a painful test.

33
Vodou Shangri-La

Spring 2005:

There had been a drought in most of Haiti for several months, so the road from Port au Prince to Thomonde was even dustier than usual. White chalk-like dust coated everything along the road as our trucks ascended *Morn Kabrit* (Goat Mountain). Emerging from a chalky fog, the children begging by the roadside looked like ghostly apparitions, their outstretched hands as webs hung on the ends of twigs. The ubiquitous dust obscured our view of the countryside below – a mixed blessing, as an unobstructed view of the road that climbed the shear face of *Morn Kabrit* was not for the faint-hearted. At the same time, the dust created a magical effect as we ascended, almost like we were passing from one world and into another.

We had left behind the frenetic activity and squalor which was Port au Prince. The dead eyes of the beggars, the pleading of the market – women, the mounds of smoldering charcoal and trash, and the cacophony of the city's millions, gave way to the desolation of *Morn Kabrit* and eventually the peace and tranquility of the mountain villages we passed through on our way to Thomonde.

It was my 103rd trip to Haiti, and approximately my sixtieth trip to Thomonde, the ultimate destination of our caravan. We had almost cancelled this particular trip, as the rebellion against Artistide had only recently succeeded, leaving anarchy on the streets of Port au Prince. That was the capital however. It would be different in Thomonde. Marie wanted us to see our community health program in action. At the same time, working with Medishare had become one of the best learning experiences possible for our student volunteers. We wouldn't want a little thing like rebellion to get in the way of their learning.

Thomonde and its people were a big reason for that success. Improbably, people of this Central Plateau commune had sought us out, invited us to come, sheltered and fed us in our early visits, and chose to make health a community priority.

In my heart, however, the joy of returning to Thomonde was not really about the program, as wonderful as it was, or my students, as enthusiastic and as hard-working as they were. No, if the truth be told, I owed the *Thomondois* more than I could ever give them. They let me have my cake and eat it too – a short flight from Miami (and admittedly a more arduous trip to Thomonde) and my life's aspirations to serve the poor were being fulfilled (too bad if it had to be for only one week at a time).

We had more than thirty doctors and medical students in tow on this particular trip. Some would stay over in *Cange* at Dr. Farmer's hospital performing surgery, while others would continue on with us to Thomonde. Once in Thomonde, we would spread out through the district, performing mobile clinics that provided screenings and preventive services each day of the week-long visit.

Our progress was slowed in *Terrier Rouge*. We had forgotten to factor in market day – an Afro-Haitian tradition that rotates markets to a different town or village each day of the week, thus expanding the opportunity of each market woman to sell her goods. What seemed like thousands of burros impeded our progress. Our drivers proceeded cautiously, not wanting to squash the eggplants, tomatoes, or zucchini arranged in neat stacks on the edge of the road.

The Artibonite River, flowing out of *Lac Peligre,* was at an all-time low. Dugout canoes lined a beach for several hundred yards from the bank – the dug-out technology taught to runaway slaves from now-vanished Arawak Indians. The road was at times desolate and at times throbbing with the life-pulse of rural Haiti. Women in peasant dresses and straw hats carried broad tan discs of cassava from markets on their heads. Children in school uniforms, men herding oxen switched their beasts on their flanks to drive them to the side of the road, out of the way of our caravan. At the headwaters of the Artibonite, women spread out their laundry to dry on cactus hedgerows while children splashed and swam in the swift river current.

The vegetation thinned as we crested above *Cange* and began our slow descent into Thomonde. Our drivers were pushing, hoping to arrive before dark, as there were no lights or shoulders on this mountainous dirt road. I too was anxious to get to Thomonde. Thinning yellow sunlight illuminated the purple grasses of the Central Plateau highlands. In this region only an occasional century plant – an algave cactus that blooms with a spectacular orange tuft of a flower once every hundred years – interrupted the windswept savannah.

Shortly thereafter, our trucks traversed the inner lip of Thomonde's gigantic caldera and descend to Thomonde proper. "Don't worry – the volcano's inactive," I dead-panned as I asked the driver to pull over at a scenic spot. The other drivers followed suit. It would be worth being a few minutes late for dinner. The students piled out of their trucks. Those with cameras took picture after picture - below us was the gigantic pie-plate-shaped caldera that geologically defined Thomonde. Having listened intently to my lesson on Hispaniola's geology on the ride up, one of the students asked "Do they have earthquakes here? If they have volcanoes, they must also have earthquakes."

"Yes, but rarely – the last was in 1847 – and not here - the fault lines lie to the north and south," I responded.

Huge royal palms, mahogany and mapou trees swayed in the breeze. The Thomonde river snaked tranquilly through the valley. Occasionally a puff of smoke would arise from a recently ignited fire. Off to the west, the sun was setting behind the cluster of mountains that contained Thomonde's most isolated village, Baille Touribe. To the north, beyond the green verge of Thomonde's defining ridge, one could see the curvature of the Earth, as well as the entire central plateau, tumbling on towards the one last mountain range between us and the sea. The sound of Vodou drums echoed from the crater below us. Thomonde – my Vodou Shangri-La.

It's not Thomonde's remoteness or isolation, nestled in the rugged mountains on the edge of the Plateau Central that so remind me of James Hilton's classic, Lost Horizon, although there are similarities. Like Shangri-La, Thomonde is virtually cut off from the outside world, except for the steady stream of Haitians traveling to Hinche and beyond on the world's worst dirt road called Route Nationale 3. Most of these travelers are unaware of the overwhelming number of Thomonde's 40,000 people who live out of sight of the highway – along the river and the mountain crests in miniscule hamlets and along the tiny footpaths that tie them together. Nor is it Thomonde's oasis-like quality, its canopy of green standing in sharp contrast to the deforested mountains and grasslands that surround it. No, it's the people and their way of life that have created this improbable paradise.

Hilton's novel is fiction, of course, while Thomonde is real – super-real, to borrow the current vogue mot from the world of Haitian art. I don't mean to romanticize Thomonde – it has all the problems one would expect from a rural community stuck in the middle of the poorest country in the Western Hemisphere. In truth, conditions were truly horrible in the early years of my visits. Rampant malnutrition, worm infestations and tuberculosis ravaged the population, not to mention the misery inflicted by mites and other skin infestations. With all that disease, it was easy to miss Thomonde's paradisiacal qualities. But, thinking back, that was the remarkable thing – in spite of those miseries, hope lived, and every once in a while, joy erupted. If Medishare, our charity, deserved any credit, it was only that it made a dent in the misery quotient, bumped up the hope factor and created a few more reasons for joy.

We descended into the principal village of Thomonde as darkness descended. Magistrat Delva, our host, greeted our arrival with a boisterous *"Byenveni!* (Welcome!) for the students and a bear-hug for Barth and me. Nimi, our cook, had a feast prepared for us, confidently expecting us at seven, exactly the time of our arrival. Our team of medical students and faculty volunteers, famished and exhausted from the seemingly interminable trip from Miami to Thomonde – two hours at the airport in Miami, three hours collecting bags, clearing customs and organizing the departure of thirty volunteers in five trucks, followed by five hours on the miserable excuse for a road that was Route Nationale 3 – devoured Nimi's feast with a vengeance, consuming within minutes her macaroni pies, beet salad, chicken Kreyol, plantains, and frosted cakes, all cooked over an open fire. Rather than complicate the feeding frenzy, knowing Nimi would not let me go hungry, I set out for an evening stroll.

Imagine a place where everyone loves you. That was Thomonde's special charm. More correctly, imagine a place where everyone loves everyone else. It was not that they just loved me and me alone, the benevolent *blan* whom their magistrat invited to bring health care to them eight years earlier. Nor was it that they loved only Medishare's volunteers, who came to them so improbably several times per year, not only caring about their health, but also jump-starting their otherwise subsistence economy with an infusion of cash and resources into the health sector. No, in spite of the poverty and poor health, from time immemorial (or at least since the village was founded in 1630), everyone in Thomonde gave love, respect and honor to everyone else they met. It was just the *Vodouisant* way.

This approach to life was everywhere evident as I took my evening walk - apparent in every interaction, group or individual, with every citizen of Thomonde, young and old, from the poorest of the poor up to the *notables* and the *magistrat*. Candles and charcoal fires were the only illumination. That particular night, the moon was new. I used a flashlight to navigate the rock and dirt streets of Thomonde, being careful not to step in mud-ruts or donkey dung, or to slip on a stone. Voices called out from the darkness as I passed. *"Respek", "Salu", "Bonswa Docte!"* to which I would respond *"Honeur… Salu, Bonswa chery."* Others passing in the street were also greeted in a similar manner. Occasionally, knots of people engaged in conversation would temporarily step forward, the men to shake my hand, the women to kiss me on both cheeks – the traditional Haitian greeting adopted from the French – all congratulating me on my safe return to Thomonde. Children vied for the opportunity to hold my hand as we walked, only to be scolded by adult passers-by if they became too boisterous or rowdy. The children and I were not the only ones holding hands – everyone walking in pairs – child-child, manwoman, man-man, and woman-woman couples – hold hands – a charming custom giving eloquent testimony that, in Thomonde at least, the biblical dictum *"Rimen vwazin-w"* (love thy neighbor) rules.

This is not to say that Thomonde doesn't have its share of domestic disputes or occasional petty theft, although Magistrat Delva has assured me repeatedly that any theft is undoubtedly perpetrated by passersthrough traveling on the national road. Crime is almost a foreign concept in Thomonde, and violent crime among the *Thomondois* was virtually absent.

When violence does intrude it was usually brought from the outside. A few months before our visit, the rebel's intent on overthrowing the government infiltrated across the Dominican border some ten miles away. They threatened our health workers, commandeered our ambulances and killed two security guards at the dam down the road at Lac Peligre. U.N. troops now assigned to Thomonde, outsiders from Brazil, were also viewed with suspicion – rumored to use their authority to have their way with the girls and women of Thomonde.

This problem had surfaced before, under the Duvalier regime, when the tentacles of dictatorship embodied in the *Ton Ton Macoutes* infiltrated every corner of Haiti, including Thomonde. Papa Doc's thugs, their white and black clothes and eyes screened by sunglasses consciously mimicking Baron Samedi, in all likelihood played a critical role in the spread of AIDS to women in the Central Plateau. No *Vodouisant* would ever exploit women like that – too much respect was owed to them, too much honor given.

Now, your average male *Thomondois* is not above flirting, seduction, or deception in matters of love, and will resort to potions and mojos (love charms). They also are willing to pay a small portion of the money they earned cutting cane across the border in the Dominican Republic for the services of the prostitutes living in the batays. But threats – covert or overt – were not part of these youths' modus operandi.

As I rounded the corner at the village square to complete the loop back to our guesthouse, after a half hour of unrelenting Thomondian politeness and hospitality, my mind drifted back again to the central paradox of Thomonde. Why, amidst all this poverty and hardship are these people so nice to everyone? Was it their upbringing? Their heritage? Their religion? All of the above? I had come to Haiti originally hoping to help ease a desperate health situation and hoping to have the opportunity to teach both Haitian doctors and my own medical students about diseases that fall under the rubric of "tropical medicine". Now, it was the Haitians that were teaching me – to a certain extent about medicine, or at least how one could be effective in a resource-poor country like Haiti – but more importantly, they were showing me how to live, perhaps even to thrive, in the most adverse of circumstances.

"Barth, I need your help in getting Janet in to see a neurologist. She's probably got a pinched nerve in her neck – hopefully she won't need your services", I whispered to my colleague and friend after I returned from my walk. That was just one of the wonderful things about Medishare – how it brought Barth, quintessential specialist and me, family doctor, together for Haiti.

After we had finished dinner the students always ask me the first night on every trip – "Dr. Fournier, tell us, what about Voodoo?"

"Well, it's late. We all need a good night's sleep and it's a complicated subject. We can't cover it all in one evening's discussion, but we can get started. *Vodou*, that's the correct name, not the English bastardization, is both a religion and a way of life. Now I hope I won't offend anyone with this discussion – how many of you are Catholic?" More than half raised their hands.

"I was born and raised Catholic also. The majority of Haitians are devout, pious Catholics. No matter what you believe about Catholicism, there's ample evidence that it succeeded in becoming the official religion of the Roman Empire, and subsequently the largest religion in the world, because of its wonderful syncretism – its ability to adapt to, absorb, and accommodate pagan traditions and beliefs. In this syncretic pantheon Athena became the Virgin Mary, Aphrodite transformed into Mary Magdalene, Apollo became Jesus, Hera became St. Anne, and so on. The same thing happened in Vodou, but with a unique Haitian twist.

"The Haitians had Catholicism forced upon them. Conditions for slaves in St. Domingue were so horrible that the average life expectancy of a slave there was measured in months, not years. Paradoxically, because of this, the majority of slaves at the time of the Haitian revolution had never lost their African roots, as usually happened to those slaves brought to America or other British colonies. So for the *Vodouisant*, the practitioner of Vodou, the *Lwa*, (from the French le roi – "the King") ("r's" in Kreyol are pronounced like "w's") their African spirits and ancestors, were more real than the saintly persona they were forced to worship under the whip and the cross.

"It amazes me how much Greco-Roman mythology survives intact in *Vodou*. Athena-the Virgin Mary is transformed into *Erzili-Freda*, (the *Lwa* the *Vodouisant* prays to when wisdom is needed) while Aphrodite-Magdalene morphs into *Erzili-Mawan* (the *Lwa* for matters of love). *La Sirene*, the mermaid, is the same siren of the Odyssey, except with a more benevolent role – she escorts the souls of the dead across the ocean, the Haitian equivalent of the River Styx, back to Guinea, their homeland and "Paradise."

"Look up into the sky!" I exclaimed, catching everyone off guard as I pointed to the stars visible through the central courtyard. "See that constellation? Gemini. Only in Vodou, they're *Marassa!* There must have been significant trade and social intercourse between the Mediterranean world and the west coast of Africa going back to ancient times – there are too many similarities to be explained only by coincidence.

Just then the sounds of *Tambou* – Vodou drums pierced the night, their staccato rhythm seemingly extracted from a vintage Tarzan movie. "Do you hear that?" I asked my students. "You can hear those drums every night here in Thomonde. It's right out of Africa and it hasn't changed for centuries. It's a culture that most Americans are, at best, only dimly aware of."

"All *Vodou* saints are called *Lwa*. Some *Lwa* represent abstractions of all aspects of human life – love and wisdom *(Erzili)*, conflict *(Ogun)*, death (Baron Samedi). They also, however, represent the souls of ancestors. All *Vodouisants* are transformed into *Lwa* (helpful spirits, available for intercession) at the moment of death. They are there always for their descendants, to whom they've passed on their wisdom and for whom they can work miracles.

The students were enthralled and eager to learn more, but it was very late. I promised them we'd revisit the subject again the next night.

Together, we'd unlock the mysteries of animism, the secrets of the zombie curse and Baron Samedi, as well as the source of the magic powers of the *bokor* and *mambo*. But it was important that we all got a good night's sleep: there was hard work to be done the following day and a long drive out to Baille Touribe, the furthest village in the commune and back.

I did, indeed, sleep well, as I invariably did in Haiti, ignorant at that time of the insidious dissolution of my wife's spinal cord, already progressing, but as yet undiagnosed. All that would change shortly after my arrival home. Perhaps Baron Samedi the Lord of the Underworld took offense to my description of him as a trickster to my students during our seminar one night there. More likely, he was really upset that he could no longer count on his quota of souls from Thomonde. Medishare was really starting to make a difference. It was a brilliant tactic on his part — it would be some time before I would either sleep as well or return to my Vodou Shangri-La again.

34
Baron Samedi

We in the west would tend to view Janet's ordeal as a losing battle against a horrible disease. *Vodouisants* would see it as "coming to the crossroads." Simply put, they see things differently than we do. Christians see the cross as a sign of redemption through suffering. In Vodou, the cross represents the intersection of life and death, past and future. In Vodou cosmology, the crossroads are guarded by Baron Samedi, Lord of the Underworld. While similar to the rulers of the dead in other religions – Pluto, Vulcan, and Satan – Samedi's persona is uniquely Vodou. This *Vodou* god, (or "*Lwa*") is often depicted in a black suit and bowler hat, brandishing rum and cigarettes with abandon, as, for his own amusement, he plays tricks on the souls of the about-to-be dead. The message to the *Vodouisant* is clear. Death was not what you imagined. Not only could you not trick death, death would invariably trick you.

Likewise, you would never catch Baron Samedi preoccupied with the great mythic stuff of other gods of the underworld, such as Pluto's obsession with Persephone – an obsession which ultimately caused the seasons to change, or Satan's rebellion, which led to the fall of Man. Rather, the Haitian Lord of the Dead is only interested in the spiritual equivalent of small change – liberating our *ti bon ange* (literally, our "good little angel"), that part of our soul that includes our consciousness and personality – from the prison of its *corpse cadaver*, its inanimate flesh. In doing so, Samedi seems akin to the Hindu god, Shiva. As Guardian of the Crossroads, he is both a destroyer and a creator. The Crossroads intersected in four directions: life and death, past and present. The Baron controls it all, leading us back and forth between this world and the realm of spirits and serving as the medium of communality between the living and the dead. That's why, at the beginning of Janet's illness, when I saw the twitches in her right forearm, I knew it was Baron Samedi at work. Every twitch seemed like a prod of the old trickster's cane in my wife's flesh. It was just too cruel a joke.

It had been the best of times for our family. Our younger daughter Suzanne was cruising through dental school. Our older daughter Adrienne transferred to a job in Orlando – much closer to our home in Miami than her previous job in Chicago. Janet taught second grade at the Cushman School, a small private school in Miami, where the headmistress called her a "legend", in recognition of her superb teaching skills. My own career in academic medicine at the University of Miami Miller School of Medicine was flourishing. So was Medishare.

Baron Samedi's chicanery was so subtle that its significance first escaped me. Janet first noted some weakness and clumsiness in her left hand during the early months of 2005. She said nothing about this annoyance, either to me or anyone else, thinking it was caused by some minor ailment. In March, when the weakness became noticeable to me, we attributed it to perhaps a pinched nerve in her neck, the result of slinging the twenty pounds of schoolbooks and papers she used in teaching over her shoulder every morning. Nevertheless, the twitches I noticed in her left arm were troubling.

I arranged an appointment for Janet with a neurologist. She was anxious about her symptoms and didn't want to go alone, so I picked her up outside of her classroom and drove her to the medical center, about five miles away. It was strange watching a colleague go through the ritual of performing a complete neurological exam on my wife. She had obvious weakness in her left hand, which could certainly be explained by a pinched nerve. Subtle weakness in other muscle groups, however, suggested that more than one nerve was involved.

The neurological examination is the pinnacle of the clinical art. It can distinguish lesions with anatomic accuracy better than a CAT scan or an MRI. As Janet's exam unfolded, the neurologist unearthed more and more bizarre findings. In addition to a distribution of weakness that suggested involvement of multiple nerves in her left arm, she had twitching (fasciculations) throughout the muscles of her left hand and arm; a sign that the connections of nerves to muscles were dying. There was subtle but definite atrophy of several muscle groups. Most alarming, however were her reflexes, which showed abnormalities not just in her left arm but all her limbs.

Now, even I was getting anxious, although I hid my anxiety behind a mask of objectivity cultivated by more than thirty years of medical practice. The neurologist was also showing visible signs of anxiety – here was the wife of a colleague with both fasciculations, a sign that the peripheral nerves were dying, and spasticity, indicating the central nervous system was involved as well. This particular constellation of symptoms suggested one disease only: Amyotrophic Lateral Sclerosis (ALS) also known as Lou Gehrig's disease – the disease that claimed the life of one of baseball's greatest players before he was forty years old. The neurologist cast furtive glances in my direction with each new finding. The violence of Janet's reflexes took even her by surprise. After the exam was completed, her doctor and I lapsed into speaking in medical jargon.

"Could this be a brachial plexopathy?" I inquired, with studied casualness.

"What's that?" asked Janet, looking dumbfounded and more frightened by the minute.

"A viral inflammation of the nerves of your shoulder," I explained, "it actually would be a good thing, because we could treat it, or it will get better eventually on its own."

"I suppose so," mumbled the neurologist, "but that wouldn't explain her long track findings" – then looking to Janet - "I mean your increased reflexes. I'd like to get an MRI of your neck....."

I agreed, although I knew that Janet would hate going through that

"While we're getting that, I added, "why not a brief trial of prednisone?"   Prednisone is the pill form of the most potent anti-inflammatory drug in our pharmacologic armamentarium. Doctors use it to treat a wide variety of disorders, from asthma to arthritis.

"I like that idea," said Janet. The subtleties of her neurological exam were lost on her, but she could see the concern on our faces and she liked the idea of trying something that might make her annoying symptoms go away. So it was agreed that we would get an MRI and try a brief trial of prednisone. She would see the neurologist again in a week, after the MRI was completed.

On the ride home, Janet peppered me with questions. "Does he think I have a brain tumor?" That was her biggest concern, followed by the possibility of multiple sclerosis.

"No, but I must admit, your exam had a few surprises...."

"Yeah! What's up with my reflexes?"

"I don't know, but you could have a bizarre complication of a viral infection…" I didn't mention the possibility of a problem even worse than a brain tumor.

Upon arriving home I offered Janet a glass of wine and checked her reflexes about a half-hour later. They were normal. Perhaps she was just over-adrenalin-ized, fearing what the neurologist might find. After two days of prednisone the twitches stopped. She felt almost euphoric. The MRI was negative. We both breathed a sigh of relief and turned our thoughts to a much-anticipated visit from Adrienne.

Everything changed in an instant a few days later. Janet, Adrienne, and I were sitting in an outdoor restaurant on a perfect April day. While waiting for our orders to arrive, Janet became fixated by the recurrence of twitching, this time in her right arm. The fixation lasted several minutes and caught both Adrienne's and my attention. For several minutes, we all sat there transfixed by the twitches and the fear etched on Janet's face. Up to that moment, Janet had lived a charmed life -- daughter and wife of doctors, mother of two beautiful and talented daughters, acclaimed teacher. Now, we all confronted the specter of her mortality.

For me, with my medical background, the twitches were most significant. This problem was no pinched nerve. We have tens of millions of muscle cells in our body, each touched by a nerve called a motor neuron that connects it to that part of our brain that decides what we want to do. If I want to point my finger, my brain sends an impulse down the motor neuron to a connection (known as a synapse) with the abductor pollicis longus muscle. As a result, my finger extends, seemingly effortlessly. The muscle cells need the connection to the motor neurons in order to survive.

If the motor neuron dies, it's corresponding muscle dies also. As it dies, it contracts one last time – an agonal fasciculation or a twitch. Although I said nothing at the time and left it to others to formally make the diagnosis, those fasciculations now on both her right and left sides told a fateful tale. Janet had Lou Gehrig's disease:

a relentless, incurable condition.

Baron Samedi had delivered me and my family to the crossroads. Janet was on a path from this world to the next. That crossing would drag on, one twitch, one motor neuron at a time, at its own inexorable pace. My crossroads would traverse a different route. I was on a path, prodded by Samedi, away from a comfortable, predictable life in Miami. Janet's struggle would ultimately transform us both into *Vodouisants.*

35
Musing on Mortality

In spite of more than thirty years of practicing medicine at one of the busiest medical centers in the nation, in spite of facing death in my patients' eyes almost daily, in spite of in-depth clinical knowledge about the process of dying, when the specter of death came calling to my family, my professional education and training failed me.

Medical science explains why we die patho-physiologically, but not metaphysically. It was my wife's tragic illness, suffering, and death which forced me to confront these metaphysical issues. My thoughts on the subject, framed by my now Haitian worldview guided me in recovering my life after Janet's death and also, coming full circle, in understanding in metaphysical terms, the meaning of Haiti's earthquake to its victims.

Modern medicine failed Janet because it has devolved from a profession, sadly, into a business -- a mirror of the modern, secular, materialistic world we live in. It did not help that Janet suffered from not just an incurable and untreatable disease but also one of the most miserable that a human being might have to endure. Her courageous struggle and medicine's (indeed, our culture's) inability either to provide comfort or answers to the questions posed by her struggle and passing forced me to seek answers not just about the meaning of her life and death, but also my own and, for that matter, the lives and deaths of all of us.

If Western medicine and culture failed me, with all my education, training, and experience in life and death issues, how much worse must it be for others who don't have this background? That thought sent me down this path, in search for the meaning of life and death - an effort to move beyond clinical and scientific knowledge to something hopefully approximating wisdom on this subject. I lived with Janet's dying for three years. Impending doom, playing out over time, gave me an anguished, palpably real experience in death and dying and ample time to reflect on its meaning. As I did,   I realized the full extent of the gift Haiti and its people have given. Their gift was an antidote to the zombie curse of our materialistic culture – one in which death is not trivialized or marginalized and one that finds meaning in all human experiences. That worldview, captured in the word *Vodouisant*, is also the key to understanding the resurrection of the Haitian people after the earthquake.

Conventional wisdom holds that the realm of science and the realm of the spirit are mutually exclusive. As the world of scientific knowledge grows, the domain of the spirit inevitably will shrink. Perhaps, ultimately, all will be explained by the random collision of molecules. As a physician steeped in the traditions of and benefits gained by the advances made by science, I'm forced to give the random molecule collision theory its due. If that's all there is, however, where do courage, devotion, imagination, and will come from? Janet and the people of Haiti, coming from completely opposite directions, showed me the answer.

Vodouisant: literally, a Vodou saint. The word seems simple enough on the surface. However, as one learns more about the exotic language of Kreyol, one realizes that seemingly simple words are layered and textured with complex history, symbolism, and meaning. Most scholars say that the English pronunciation "voodoo" is derived from the West African word *"Vodou,"* meaning "spirit." Ginette the psychiatry resident who first taught me about Vodou claimed the word was simply the Kreyol pronunciation of "vieux deux", the "old gods" in French – referring to the spirits of the forest that were worshiped in secret by slaves brought to Haiti from West Africa – or "vous deux" ("you two"), signifying the shared humanity of Vodou practitioners. Likewise "Sant", often assumed to be the Kreyol pronunciation for the French (or English) word "saint", is more likely derived from the word meaning "healthy" (sant).

The association between healthiness and holiness can be traced back linguistically to antiquity – for examples, saintliness and sanitation have the same root in Latin, while holiness, wholesome and holistic all spring from holos in ancient Greek. A *Vodouisant*, therefore, is much more than a practitioner of an ancient exotic religion. A *Vodouisant* is also a practitioner of a way of life that is simultaneously holy, healthy, and whole - the antithesis of the way most modern westerners live.

The apparent vagaries and contradictions of Haitian culture are frequently misunderstood. Americans, for example, may envision the voodoo of Hollywood stereotype - sticking pins in dolls to inflict pain or misfortune on one's enemy. Voodoo has become a pejorative term, as in "voodoo economics" or "voodoo science". Indeed, as I began to think about how to tell this story, I chose *Vodouisant* as a way of representing Janet as a "voodoo saint" – an unorthodox person who led a good life in spite of not adhering to the tenets of a formal religion.

To understand Vodou, one must first understand Haitians and their culture. There's no doubting the stark contrast with American culture.

Haiti's cultural roots in Africa, coupled with an isolation spawned by the international reaction to the only slave rebellion ever to succeed, created an utterly unique enclave. After all, the human species started in Africa, and Haitians are Africans transplanted in the New World. Haiti's escape from colonialism make it one of the last repositories of our essential pre-modern humanity – more so than modern African republics, forced by European powers to accept the veneer of western languages, customs and dress.

Central to this Haitian world-view is its ancient, animist, genius of a religion called *Vodou*. If one defines religion as a set of beliefs and values that provide an individual or community with a framework to understand the great mysteries of life, *Vodou* is at least as much a religion as all the others. In fact, viewed objectively, it arguably has some superior features.

With its origins in animism, it qualifies as one of the oldest religions on the planet. In many ways, it's among the purest – uncluttered with hierarchy, dogma, decadence, or corruption. The central tenets of *Vodou* – the respect shown to ancestors, the old, and children, the merged roles of priests, physicians and *Vodouisants* themselves and the search for meaning in everything – are poorly understood or purposefully distorted by its traditional western counterparts. Then there's the fascinating syncretism of *Vodou*, similar to early Roman Catholicism – its ability to marry and merge myths from Africa, Catholicism, and Greco-Roman paganism. This syncretism makes *Vodou* a truly ecumenical faith. In fact, most Haitians practice some other Christian denomination and don't see a conflict. "Haiti is 85 percent Catholic, 15 percent Protestant and 100 percent Vodou" is how my Haitian friends explain this paradox. As a way of life, even an atheist, apostate, agnostic, or secular scientist can practice it. All of these modern, western variations on the theme of materialism must eventually grapple with the issue of spirit, and Vodou, at its heart, is about spirit -- spirit and our relationships to one another. So Vodou must be understood as being radically different from its stereotypes.

Take the zombie myth. The stereotype is an image of a lumbering, brain-dead, walking cadaver hell-bent on murder and mayhem. In actuality, the zombie myth in Haiti is really about death and resurrection, freedom and slavery. *Zombé* in Kreyol means "like a shadow." The victim of the curse appears dead and is buried only to be exhumed by the *Vodou* priest, administered an antidote and enslaved in a shadow-like state until penance is served. While the Catholics talk about the concept of death and resurrection, the slavery of sin and the freedom of redemption, *Vodouisants* actually live them. Thus is the power of Vodou.

Vodou is also about rebellion, originally a rebellion against the French and their particularly cruel brand of slavery. Now, we slaves of modernity, both in medicine and general, need a rebellion, to shake us out of our zombiesque complacency. Embracing materialism and religion simultaneously and seeing no conflict, we are technologically brilliant yet simultaneously unwise. We are frequently suspicious of those searching for metaphysical answers. As a defense mechanism, we minimize, discount, dismiss, and downgrade those alternative worldviews. We ridicule them with stereotypes. We do what we've done to Vodou.

36
Ancestor Worship

Looking back, it's amazing how much my ancestors had in common with my newfound friends in rural Haiti – the primacy of family, the large size of most families, the reverence held for children, old folks and ancestors, not to mention a syncretic version of Catholicism centering on veneration of saints. At the heart of all these similarities, in spite of huge geographic and ethnic differences, were the core values forged in the face of collapsing rural economies. It was the collapse of rural economies that brought my Italian and French-Canadian grandparents to the United States, and it was the collapse of Haiti's rural economy that drove hundreds of thousands of poor Haitians to give up their birthright of land and attempt survival, either by squatting in slums of the capital like Cité Soleil, or by risking the crossing of the Windward Passage in rickety wooden boats to Miami. Ancestor worship (it's actually reverence for ancestors rather than worshipping them) and supplication to *Lwa*/saints are among the fundamental tenets of Vodou. In retrospect, my whole family were *Vodouisants* of sorts from the beginning.

When I was eight or nine, my French-Canadian memé (grandmother) gave me a book entitled The Lives of the Saints. It contained about twelve chapters, each starting with an artist's rendition of a saint, followed by an inspiring recounting of the saint's life. Curiously, it ignored the saints and martyrs of the early Church, focusing instead on saints from medieval and modern times. Thinking back, although the book was written in English, its author was probably French-Canadian, for the lives of St. Louis and Jeanne D'Arc were prominently featured, along with the Jesuits martyred by the Iroquois. Also included in this eclectic edition were St. Ignatius of Loyola, St. Dominic, and St. Francis of Assisi.

The Lives of the Saints soon became my favorite book. I read it again and again — usually one chapter at a time, followed by hours of day - dreaming, meditation, and contemplation on the saint's picture. *Vodouisants* also contemplate upon pictures of saints, for the same reason their medieval counterparts meditated on stain glass windows — they couldn't read and the pictures told the story. The story for Haitians, of course would have a Vodou twist — their saints would have dual persona, both Catholic and Vodou. Pictures of St. Patrick driving the snakes out of Ireland are revered in Haiti — not because St. Patrick himself was a runaway slave (a fact that most Haitians or Irish are not aware of), but because while we see St. Patrick, they see *Damballah*, the snake *Lwa*. *Damballah* – Dam the African word for snake and Allah the Arabic word for God, is the same abstraction the Greek and Romans embodied in our icon of the medical profession, the Caduceus — a symbol of power, health and healing. These connections would become apparent to me only decades later.

Other boys my age emulated war heroes, professional athletes, comic book heroes. I, like a Vodou acolyte, aspired to sainthood. Of course, this avocation to holiness occurred well before I entered puberty. I was then unaware of the importance the Church placed on the chasteness of its would-be saints. My nine-year-old mind saw no contradiction between the military virtues of Sts. Louis, Jeanne, and Ignatius, and the gentleness and humility of St. Francis. It was simple, really. Why wouldn't one want to grow up to be like one of these holy people?

There were also real-life saints in my life to emulate. Memé herself was pious enough, believing intensely in the miraculous possibilities of cure through pilgrimage, particularly to the shrine of Ste. Anne de Beaupré, northeast of Québec City. Her piety paled in comparison, however, to Nana, my Italian grandmother. It was not by accident that my grandparents' house – a double-decker on Hutchinson Street, in Revere, Massachusetts – was just across the street from St. Anthony's church. A marvel of Italian Romanesque architecture, the church was nestled among the tenements of Revere, which, along with East Boston, Chelsea, and Boson's North End, comprised one of the largest Italian ghettoes of the New World. St. Anthony's was at the center of my grandmother's life. Every morning of her life she attended mass. Just like the Haitians, even when she wasn't in church, she was always praying – not to God the Father, mind you, but to the saints, chief of whom, in my grandmother's pantheon, was the Virgin Mary. It was as if, being a mother herself, the Virgin would understand my grandmother's needs even more than God himself. There was never any shortage of possible beneficiaries for her prayers, what with eleven children, (seven of them daughters), and grandchildren seemingly more numerous than the stars in the sky.

Papa, my grandfather, with his penchant for his home-made wine and a seemingly perpetual irascibleness towards at least one of his sons-in-law on any given day, maintained a St. Joseph-like devotion to the protection of his family. The ultimate father-as-bread-winner, he would trudge every day, regardless of the vagaries of New England weather, five miles each way down the Lynn Marsh Road from his home on Hutchinson St. to his job at the General Electric plant in Lynn. He never missed a day of work in fifty years. Even during the Depression, he always worked.

We visited my grandparents' home every Sunday – each visit part rough-and-tumble games with my cousins, part visit to the family shrine, and part Italian peasant feast, complete with seductive sips of my grandfather's wine. Homemade ravioli were spread out to dry on my grandparents' bed under the watchful eyes of the large statue of the Virgin Mary that hovered on a platform above it, bedecked with palm-fronds and votive candles.

Later, each Sunday, Nana's ravioli, along with a host of other delicacies, would be consumed by her extended family at the dining room table, behind which hung a copy of DaVinci's The Last Supper. Portraits of other saints and the Holy Family graced every room in the house. It was a holy house, really, to the extent that I even wondered why my Nana even bothered crossing the street to go to church, other than the fact that the Church mandated it.

Saintly behavior was even expected from us grandchildren – any fall from grace during our Sunday visits was quickly reversed by a variety of penances, ranging from a burst of epithets in Italian (inscrutable but usually effective) to an occasional rap from Nana's wooden spoon or a wallop from Papa's leather shaving strap. The Haitians also believe in the strict discipline of children, a custom at times confused with child abuse here in America.

If discipline alone were not enough to inspire piety, we received weekly reinforcement in the confessional on Saturdays and from the pulpit on Sundays. Aspiration to a holy life was a key factor in my choice to become a physician, a calling which I chose shortly after receiving The Lives of the Saints. What better way for a bright young boy with skills in science to serve God than to heal the sick? Haitians are equally as pious – frequent attending two services each Sunday. Of course, one of the services might be Vodou.

My father worked three jobs to support us while my mother stayed at home to raise what eventually became a brood of six. Most working class Haitians I know also work several jobs. I was the oldest, and my parents, after considerable angst, decided not to risk my chances for advancement in life on the public high school of my hometown, Peabody. They enrolled me in a newly opened Catholic high school, Bishop Fenwick, named after the second bishop of Boston. The difficulty of that decision was eased somewhat by the fact that, as a new school, its tuition was ridiculously low - $125 a year! – otherwise, a parochial education would have been beyond my parents' means. Similarly, when it became time for college, there was only one choice: Merrimack College, founded by the Augustinian Fathers in 1947, in North Andover, a brief sixteen-mile commute from my home, up Route 114. Merrimack's tuition was also a bargain, less than $2,000 per year. Even that financial burden was eased by scholarships, including one from the Revere chapter of the Sons of Italy. By the time I entered college, I was thoroughly indoctrinated in Catholic dogma, had seriously considered a vocation in the priesthood and had decided I would most likely spend my life as a medical missionary.

Merrimack's administration hoped to make the newly-founded college competitive with other New England Catholic liberal arts colleges – the next Boston College or Holy Cross. As a consequence, in addition to a full plate of pre-med courses, I was also required to take a complete liberal arts curriculum, including at least one course per semester in philosophy or theology. The result was a challenging but superb curriculum that taught me at least as much in the realm of liberal arts as it did the traditional pre-med science courses. The Augustinians hoped that this heavy dose of philosophy, theology, history and other liberal arts would shore up the intellectual underpinnings of their students' faith. In my case, at least, they would have to be content with mixed results.

On the one hand, the course on the life of Jesus was truly inspiring, even outdoing the stories in Lives of the Saints. What a role model the historical Jesus was – humble pacifist, iconoclastic anti-hypocrite, and ultimate martyr! The course on comparative religions (taught by a rabbi,

I might add) was also enlightening, highlighting the shared themes of all great religions. However (and Catholic educators everywhere take note), the course on the history of the Church had just the opposite of its intended effect – after reviewing the two-thousand-year history of the Church, with all its warts – the scandals, schisms, and saints who turned out not to even exist – it took an act of faith to still be faithful.

This intellectual sparring would not, however, have affected my aspirations to sainthood if fate had not intervened. I didn't know it then, but know now, that even this turn of events was Samedi's work. My faith in God – at least the God of Roman Catholicism – received a crippling blow when my father died suddenly one week after his fortieth birthday. His death left my mother a widow at age thirty nine and me, at age eighteen, the de facto father to my younger brothers and sister. Ironically, I was reading Albert Camus' The Plague at the time. Here was Dr. Rieux's fictional question to Father Paneloux made real, in the anguish that I saw in the faces of my family – if there really is a loving and merciful God, then why should the innocent suffer? This would not be the last time I would need to face this question in my life.

Throughout the rest of my college years I continued going through the motions of my faith, but my father's death and my anger about it brought down the whole Catholic world of theology and dogma like a house of cards. Yet I still wanted to live the life of a saint – not necessarily an ascetic life, but at least one dedicated to doing good. It became the big philosophical question in my life, for which it would take forty years to find an answer – in a godless world, what was the point of altruism?

My first week in medical school our dorm proctor had gathered all of the first year students together and counseled, "You're in now, the hardest part is over and your courses are all pass-fail. Each of you needs to find something outside of medicine, be it animal, vegetable, or mineral, to sink your passion into. It will help you keep your sanity and humanity." I took him at his word and took it one step further. I chose two passions. Janet and I met that same night. We soon became inseparable, going every evening for dinner at the Boston City Hospital cafeteria (for medical students, all you could eat for .50¢) and afterwards to my dorm room to "study." During the summer we would escape to her parents' cottage on Cape Cod. There, I taught myself sailing on her father's day-sailor. Sailing became my second passion.

Any last hopes on the part of my mother or my grandparents that I might rediscover my faith were dashed by Janet. She was Jewish, you see, and of no mindset to deal with tortured Catholic angst. She was also impossibly cute – a petite size 2, and, for lack of a better word, sexy. Of course, the rumors that I had heard from my friends at college – that Jewish girls were sexier, or at least more interested in sex than their Catholic peers – only enhanced her allure. As our relationship heated up, I dropped all pretense of practicing Catholicism.

She was not just from a different religion – she was from an entirely different social class. Her father was a pediatrician and she grew up in the well-to-do Boston suburb of Framingham. If ever there was an example of the expression "opposites attract," we were it.

It was the late sixties – Dr. King and two Kennedys had been assassinated and President Nixon was soon to invade Cambodia. A commitment to social justice, civil rights, and a firm opposition to the war in Vietnam had already filled the void in my life created by the abandonment of formal religion. In particular, I had committed my career to bringing health care to the poor. Janet had much less interest in these causes than I did. To her credit, though, she tolerated my passion for all this and ever joined me at rallies and protests.

Her first visits with my family were studies in bilateral culture shock. My brothers wondered why she couldn't hit a baseball, while my sister seethed at the usurper who was threatening to claim her surrogate father. Janet, on her part, had never experienced anything like our large family get-togethers, filled with chaos and congeniality, nor could she relate to my mother or grandmother's saintly devotions. She was particularly appalled that there were seven of us living in a house with only one bathroom – it was unfathomable to her that one would have to share a bathroom or wait one's turn. My grandfather died a few months after we met – she stood in awe at the graveside as my grandmother cried out my grandfather's name – seventy years of shared life not blunting, but rather fueling, her passionate grief. Such things were not done in her family.

We married during my last year in medical school and soon discovered the art of marital compromise. I ranked Miami's Jackson Memorial Hospital as my first choice for residency and matched. For me, it was a busy city hospital serving the poor of Miami. For Janet, it was Miami, perpetually warm and exotic. It was clear to me that my dreams of working in some place like Africa or Haiti would never fly with Janet, but she was also willing to compromise. After residency, I volunteered for the National Health Service Corps, assigned to rural Virginia. As much as I loved it there – treating all patients from all walks of life regardless of their ability to pay – she hated it: too rural, too "southern" (her code-word for socially conservative), no shopping. So after my two-year commitment expired, we compromised again and returned to Miami, where I accepted a position on the faculty at the University of Miami School of Medicine. By that time, dreams of sainthood were long forgotten. Given our teaching hospital's nature as a county hospital, however, at least my job afforded me the opportunity to maintain my commitment to the poor. At the same time, Janet worked hard to ensure that my sense of social responsibility didn't infringe to any large degree on our family life.

In addition to her sex appeal, the other thing so alluring about Janet in the early days of our relationship was her carefreeness. I had a tendency to take everything too seriously. Janet's personality was a good antidote for that seriousness. So for seven years, from the first week of medical school until the birth of our first daughter, we were inseparable, except for work, passionate and devoted to one another. That all changed drastically when Janet assumed the responsibilities of motherhood. Suddenly, she was the more serious one and I took a back seat to the raising of our daughters and later to her commitment to teaching. In short, we grew apart, living almost separate lives, although we shared a common roof and devotion to our children and families. My work in Haiti proved a constant source of friction… Janet resented the time I spent there and viewed it as a dangerous place where I might get killed. Years passed. Tomorrow and tomorrow crept its petty pace, until the day that Baron Samedi reappeared, ready to claim Janet prematurely.

37
Therapeutic Nihilism

"We've been waiting for you," my colleague Wally said as I came into his office. A neurologist, department chairman and resident expert on neuromuscular disorders, Wally had just completed a "second opinion" examination of Janet. I was coming to pick her up.

"I didn't want to have to repeat myself," he said.

I apologized for being late. He seated me in the Chippendale chair next to Janet. I took her hand.

"You have Lou Gehrig's Disease," he said to her. "I hate to be the bearer of bad news, but there can be no doubt, based upon your exam and EMG findings. You'll develop progressive muscle weaknesses and spasticity." After a pause, he added, almost as an afterthought, "If there's good news in all of this, you'll have no pain with this, and sphincter muscles are not affected…"

My eyes focused on Janet. Janet's jaw clenched, her grip on the arm of the chair tightened, and the hairs on the back of her neck stood on end. A long, uncomfortable silence ensued.

"How much time do I have?" Janet asked.

"Average life expectancy from day of diagnosis – which would be today, I might add – is two to five years." Janet's jaw clenched so tightly that it sent waves of fasciculatory spasms through the rest of the muscles in her face. I was hoping some wisdom would follow.

"Of course, there is no cure," he continued, "but there are things that you can do – should you have difficulty breathing, we have a small machine to assist you," Janet sat and smiled at him impassively. "And there may be nutrition issues."

"I don't want a respirator and I don't want a feeding tube." Janet interrupted. "I'll take a powder long before that. Do you give sleeping pills?"

The chair ignored Janet's inquiry into euthanasia, and continued on about his ALS Center and all the services it could provide. He also asked us for hair samples – there was some evidence in mice that a certain neurohormone found in soil bacteria could be what triggered the disease.

"Otherwise," he added dryly, "we're pretty much in the dark about this disease, both in terms of cause and cure."

So much for wisdom.

Janet's body language imperceptibly softened when he mentioned possible treatments. Could he give her prescriptions, she enquired. She would start that evening. I was more skeptical. One of the medicines he recommended, Riluzole, sounded like Aricept, a pill touted for treatment of the early stages of Alzheimer's disease. No doctor treating Alzheimer's seriously believed the drug had any real effect. Faced, however, with the prospect of therapeutic nihilism, what could I say?

We made small talk for a couple of minutes and we thanked him for squeezing us in before Janet's vacation. The encounter ended with a somewhat contrived hugging exercise, at his insistence – first he with each of us and then us with each other.

Janet sat in silence on the ride home. She went straight to our bedroom, removed her clothes, and climbed under the bedcovers. The muscles of her arm were twitching like a can of nightcrawlers. She asked that I join her in bed and we embraced – for the first time in a long time. She placed her head on my shoulder, sobbed a sob or two, and, to my surprise, was soon asleep.

Hours passed and it was pitch dark when she finally awoke. The total darkness coupled with the warmth under the covers and the silence except when we spoke created the impression that our bodies didn't exist, that we were just two souls talking.

"I hate him!" she exclaimed suddenly, with her voice slightly raised.

"You just want to shoot the messenger. Someone had to break the bad news."

"I don't want to die, Arthur, but I don't want anything to do with respirators or feeding tubes."

"You don't have to. You're in charge. Only your wishes count as to how you want to be treated."

"I don't know how to explain this to our family. This will kill my father... I'll need your help."

"We'll do it together."

"You'll need to change your plans about Haiti. You need to come home to the Cape with me. I can't do this alone." Prior to our visits with the neurologists, I was planning on going to Haiti in June with Medishare. Janet planned to spend that time with her family in Cape Cod. It pained me to hear that I'd have to give up my trip to Haiti. I realized this was not the only trip I would miss. I would have to cancel most, if not all, trips until Janet's illness played itself out. I had visited Haiti over hundred times since I started working there a decade before. The trips had become simultaneously an opportunity to do good and teach, not just about medicine, but also life. Haiti served as an antidote to the materialism I found so discouraging in Miami, even in our own lives, as well as a balm for my troubled spirit and an opportunity to see the world from a whole different perspective. My times in Haiti had become the most meaningful experiences in my life.

"Okay, I will."

The words stuck somewhat in my throat, but I knew I had no choice.

"Come on, get up. Let's go over to some restaurant on South Beach. I'll treat you to supper."

38
A Day at the Beach

By October 2005, Janet's disease had progressed to a point that her left hand was essentially useless. Subtle but definite weakness was also beginning to show in her right hand, but she was determined to keep teaching and continued to drive herself each day the short twenty blocks to her school. The teaching assistant the school assigned to her to help with routine activities proved invaluable in her struggle to continue working as long as possible.

At an alarming pace, Janet became increasingly dependent on me for all of the household duties, duties I had taken for granted that she would always be able to do. Janet, for some time, resisted bringing in home healthcare workers. They would be expensive and she didn't like having possibly untrustworthy strangers alone with her in our home. By default, I became her caregiver. I quickly became aware of many things about progressive paralysis that they never taught us in medical school -- just how dependent we are on our non-dominant hand and fingers to complete mundane tasks, such as tying one's shoes or pulling up a zipper. Before I knew it, I was spending four to five hours each day dressing and undressing Janet, assisting in her ablutions, cooking, cleaning up after meals, shopping— all the things that Janet had done before as a matter of course.

For many years, Janet had been my harshest critic. Ironically, her illness would draw us together again. She joked to our daughters that I was actually becoming a saint. How ironic that it would take Janet's mortal illness to resurrect my childhood aspiration to sainthood--or perhaps that was just another of Samedi's tricks. But our daughters passed on advice they received from their ALS support groups – caregivers need support too, at least in the form of a little "time-out" now and then. Thus, it was decided that my sister, who also lives in Miami, would stay with Janet on alternate Sundays, allowing me to go sailing.

When we moved to Florida, I invested my first paycheck as an intern ($400) into a ten-foot sailing dinghy, which I kept chained to a palm tree behind our apartment on Key Biscayne. It proved to be a perfect antidote to the stresses of internships and residency. While sleep deprivation and long hours on-call morphed many of my fellow interns into zombies, I spent my precious free time sailing on Biscayne Bay. Janet accompanied me frequently back then, but after the birth of our daughters, her interest rapidly waned. She wouldn't admit it, but as she grew older, the leaning of any sailboat into the wind frightened her to the point of panic. For many years, therefore, I had sailed without her -- sometimes with our daughters, but usually alone.

The solitude of solo sailing gave me ample time to contemplate the twists and turns in our lives, how different we were in the beginning, and how we drifted apart. Those reflections reminded me of the philosophical conflicts still unresolved from my youth — the clash of values that we put on hold to make our relationship work. I tried to make sense of it all- to sort things out why I was the person I was and led the life I did. It was, I had to admit, a schizophrenic life of altruism at work and materialism at home.   Invariably, the outside world would intervene. A gust of wind, a threatening downpour, or a close encounter with a careening power boater invariably broke these unhurried and meandering thoughts.

With Janet's diagnosis, these unsettled thoughts felt more urgent. With each passing day, with each new infirmity, the pressure mounted. If our unresolved relationship issues were at the root of all these conflicts, perhaps now was the time to bring some healing to us both.   One Sunday in October, Mother Nature finally helped me chart a course through this existential morass.

Late in the morning the wind died and I was forced to run the small diesel engine of "First Star", the twenty-five-foot sloop I had purchased two years before. Nothing interrupts the solitude of sailing more than the chug-a-chug of a diesel engine and the smell of its exhaust, so I abandoned my plans for sailing that afternoon and set course for the beach. My usual sailing ground, the northern part of Biscayne Bay, is separated from the Atlantic by a narrow strip of land – a sandbar, really – just wide enough for a public park and marina on one side of the road and a beach on the other. As I maneuvered my sailboat next to one of the docks, I was greeted by a group of ever-hungry pelicans, waddling and squawking as I secured the boat with lines at the bow and stern. After locking the companionway, I grabbed a towel and my lunch, and then crossed the road in search of a quiet place to sit.

Quiet is a relative term on Haulover Beach on Sundays. There were probably more than a thousand of my fellow human beings there that day, the crowd displaying the entire spectrum of humanity – a kaleidoscope of ages, shapes, colors and languages - reflecting the enormous diversity of Miami, as well as its desirability as a tourist destination. All these people had come there on that Sunday to share one thing – the simple pleasure of a perfect afternoon by the sea. The beach was so crowded that I almost decided to return to my boat, convinced that the solitude I was seeking would not be possible that day. As I scanned the crowd, however, something about the scene intrigued me. The crowd displayed a universal carelessness rare in city life. For a few short hours the beach-goers would put aside the trappings of "modern" civilization and kick back and enjoy a primal moment. It was this carefree, naturalness which had first so attracted me to Janet. Over time, however, our lives had become complicated by the increasing demands of our professional lives as well as the demands of raising our children. Carefree moments together became rare. Moreover, as she grew older, Janet became more conservative and cautious. It was as if caution would somehow protect her from the vagaries of fate.

I had witnessed this same sort of primal joy many times on my frequent trips to Haiti. There, it had struck me as even more remarkable, as it played against a backdrop of abysmal poverty. It all came back to me in a rush – the laughter of the children frolicking naked in the Thomonde River, the squeals of delight in the soccer games at the orphanage Bercail Bon Berger or the orgiastic Kris of a Vodou ceremony. It was a strange paradox, really, its contradictions as vivid as any in that nation of extremes. In Haiti, people were joyful when they weren't miserable. In America, many are so anesthetized by our generally comfortable lives that moments of joy are compartmentalized into special events – a child's birthday party, a wedding anniversary, a day at the beach.

Each of us needs moments of joy, for they fuel hope, illusory or not, that life is worth living. We are a species that survives on hope. We have the intelligence to recognize our ultimate fate, but we must hope that the joys of life outweigh its pain. Without hope, families and communities would dissolve, societies would crumble, and people would simply stop reproducing. In short, our species would become extinct.

Of the thousand people on the beach that day, assuredly, many had problems equal or greater than mine, but given a few moments of pleasure, such as this sunny afternoon by the shore, they were able to carry on. The rest relied on unprovable and unrealistic assumptions – that they'd live to an advanced old age; that they would not become incapacitated by disease; that suffering was something fate reserved for someone else. Like most of us,

Janet had always assumed that a long and happy life was a given, an entitlement, if you will. Given the level of material comfort and technical wizardry in this country, that expectation was quite understandable. In reality, however, a long and happy life for us is, at best, a probability. In Janet's case, her odds of having that entitled life seemed good, thanks to the accident of her birth into a family of means, with a history of longevity, and in a rich and powerful country. But Baron Samedi had decided to teach us this lesson, a lesson learned by every Vodouisant in Haiti. In reality, the survival of no one can be guaranteed, nor should we expect a life without suffering. Janet's vision of life, including a successful career, the vicarious enjoyment of our daughters' achievements, and a quiet death in her sleep at age of one hundred was an illusion.

Baron Samedi's message to Janet was clear. Was there a message for me as well? At age fifty eight, I was about to become a widower. I was in good health and in relatively good shape. I was a physician and a tenured professor. I was almost famous and almost wealthy. The temptations of a hedonistic life were abundantly displayed before me on the beach. "Why not seize the day? You never know how many days you have left. Is that what you're trying to tell me, Samedi?" I asked.

Many conscientious clinicians were "dropping out" – retiring early or seeking other lines of work. Perhaps it was time to coast. After all, I was a mere five years from early retirement. Then, immediately, I realized I was fooling myself. Sure, I enjoyed the pleasures of life. I had no interest in becoming an ascetic. Yet I had always wanted more. I enjoyed my work – it gave me, beyond pleasure, a profound sense of satisfaction. It was one of two things that gave meaning to my life – the other being my family.

Perhaps the lesson of Janet's illness was there was no meaning in life – that it's all, at best explained by the random collision of molecules and at worst, the evil chicanery of the gods. Somehow, however, I could just not accept that. As a child I had aspired to sainthood. Now, it appeared that I would most likely outlive my wife. I would have the freedom to pursue the ideals of altruism and service to the poor which had galvanized me in my youth. But why? Janet's suffering rekindled the metaphysical angst that had accompanied my father's death.

Over the years, I had lost my moral compass. I had become an apostate and an agnostic. If there were no God or if the gods were all tricksters like Baron Samedi, what possible rationale could there be for living the life of a saint? For that matter, forget anything even approaching sainthood. In a godless, materialistic world, why bother being moral, ethical or even, just plain good?

Science had taught me too many facts that contradicted the dogma I had learned as a child. Furthermore, I had never forgiven the God of that childhood for my father's death. Now he had Janet's fate to answer for. No, I would find no answers in the pleasures of hedonism or the formal teachings of the Church. I had lived with an agnostic for my entire adult life and a lot of that her rationalism had rubbed off on me.

I had been following the media debate over intelligent design - the latest attempt to teach Creationism in public schools. "Amazing," I thought. "Not one shred of evidence in support of the Biblical interpretation of creation, and vast amounts of evidence supporting evolution, yet, astoundingly, almost two centuries after Darwin figured out the origin of our existence, the majority of Americans still clung to belief in creation."

Why? Because creation implies a Creator – the ultimate unprovable assumption – the omniscient Being with the power to punish evil and reward good with life everlasting. People don't want to abandon the idea of a Creator because that's the rationale for leading a moral life, at least for most of us in the West. Watching Janet lose her soul one motor neuron at a time convinced me that there's no reality to the idea of eternal life. If you want to know what it will be like after you die, try to remember back before you were born. It's the same nothingness. Yet, within the confines of our mortality, there was no denying the realm of spirit – all those intangibles, those values like courage and live I witnessed growing in Janet daily.

Perhaps, if there were a God, that was part of the plan all along. If we knew for sure that God existed, moral choices would be easy. At the same time, their value of those choices would be discounted. As I could see no way around this contradiction, the best path seemed to be to keep an open mind about all things metaphysical and see some semblance of truth based on one's knowledge and experience – to leave the door cracked open for God to slip back in, just in case he's out there. There just so much we don't know, and will probably never know, no matter how much science advances.

As the day progressed a light breeze began to stir. Instead of resuming my sail, however, I remained on the beach, ruminating. Just then, a flock of pelicans, perhaps the same ones that had greeted me earlier, glided overhead in perfect v-formation. On land, these birds seemed absurdly awkward, waddling, and squatting guano, and tucking their exaggerated beaks tightly against their chests to avoid scraping them on the ground. In flight, however, they were a marvel, circling and stalling at the sight of a fish below the surface of the water, then diving and deftly snaring their prey. Watching this aerial ballet unfold before me, the insight I had been seeking revealed itself. Suddenly, the paradox of pelicans made everything clear.

Yes, there was intelligent design, and it came from our genes, honed and perfected by the need of each species to survive. For millions of years mindless microbes reproduced, gradually evolving into more complex forms, driven by what Darwin called "natural selection", what Mendel proved to be genes, and what we now know as DNA. The AIDS virus was a perfect example of this genetic intelligence - flourishing and replicating by the trillions, exploiting the human species' sex drive, immune systems, and social order, all to its terrible advantage. All life on earth was comprised of individual experiments in survival value, a mixing and matching of physical and, in more recently evolved animals, mental traits designed to discover which of the myriad combinations of DNA sequences gave the best competitive advantage in a certain environment. The same genes that made the pelicans ugly and awkward on land allowed them to flourish gracefully in the air and sea.

Now there was a time in the history of life on Earth when immortality was possible – the simple organisms that reproduced by binary fission replicated themselves exactly for eons. With these organisms possessing only vegetative functions, however, this immortality meant nothing, however. The evolution of sex, however, changed everything. Sex and death became the inextricably intertwined forces propelling the evolution of all higher species. Mortality became the price all living organisms had to pay in order to evolve to higher forms. Death and sex and evolution had chiseled out these marvelous creatures gliding before me.

We human beings are like those pelicans – genetically engineered evolutionary trade-offs, in certain settings absurd and in others sublime, honed individually and collectively to fill a certain ecological niche. The trade-offs for walking upright were but one example – it freed our hands to make tools, which in turn added a further value to the need to evolve intelligence. At the same time, childbirth became more difficult and we became slower than many of our four-footed enemies. Mothers needed to carry and feed their young until they learned to walk. Of necessity, we evolved as social animals.

The emergence of human intelligence, however, changed the rules of evolution. Decisions we make, individually and collectively, knowingly or unknowingly, affect our survival not only as individuals but also as a species. The pleasure experienced by an individual, so obvious here on the beach, must be balanced by the knowledge that we are imperfect, interdependent creatures constantly struggling to find ways to exist in an imperfect world. With intelligence, every human needs not only to survive but to flourish. Is the hope for moments of joy and pleasure for our children and ourselves that keeps us going. Without that hope, the human race is doomed.

It is obvious how we evolve traits that help the individual survive – the ability to produce adrenalin in times of danger is a simple example. Less apparent, but equally as real, is the need to evolve traits to help our species survive and flourish. This was the biological heart of ethics. Attributes that help both the individual and the species survive and flourish were certainly good things. Conversely, things that threaten both the individual and our species were categorically bad. Ethical dilemmas arose when we're forced to choose between our own survival, the survival of others, or our species.

We have evolved as frail organisms with a long period of dependence upon our parents for food, shelter, and safety. Perhaps that is where the altruism gene arose, from the sacrifices made to raise our children, in hope for a better life for them. In fact, there's some recent scientific evidence for a physiologic mediation for altruism related to hormones related to nursing. The hormones that give mothers pleasure when they nurse babies also rise when we help on another. Once present in our gene pool, this altruism gene (or genes) would prove to have survival value in other realms as well. Individually frail, our genes discovered that we needed to help each other.

To be sure, Altruism was only one of several socially positive gene clusters that fostered our survival. Others certainly included language, reason, and courage, in fact, all the intangibles that the ancients, lacking our knowledge of evolution and genetics, canonized as "soul". These socially positive genes need not be present in every individual but must exist in a significant number of people – a critical mass – if we are to survive. Furthermore, there's a spectrum of presence of these genes in the general population. Not everyone will have the courage to fall on a grenade to save his trench mates or the intelligence to work through the relationship between matter, energy, and the speed of light. Some will, however, and we're all the better for it.

My thoughts returned to Haiti and the joy and hope displayed by otherwise desperate people fighting nearly insurmountable obstacles, in one of the world's poorest countries. That joy and hope arose from the practice of Vodou, a syncretic religion happily coexisting alongside Christianity. Its principles – veneration of ancestors, healthy and holy living, honor and respect to fellow Vodouisants – all have strong survival value. These principles help to make life bearable – even joyful – under intolerable conditions. If that weren't enough, Vodouisants find meaning in everything that happens in life. That meaning was what I was searching for, and perhaps had just found.

At the same time, Janet's approaching death forced my mind back to questions of immortality. She, of course, didn't believe in life after death. The faith of her ancestors, Judaism, is silent on the subject. The faith of my ancestors, Catholicism certainly does. Official Church dogma would damn her and all non-Catholics to Hell. Would a loving God really be so dogmatic, particularly given all the good she's done in life and how much she suffered? It's hard to really know what Vodou really teaches about life after death. Vodouisants clearly believe in it, in fact elevating their dead to the status of Ti Lwa – family saints. But the nature of that existence is blurry – it seems to be dependent on the veneration offered by one's family – no veneration, no afterlife. So Vodou's view of mortality is in a certain sense more realistic. Perhaps being kept alive in the memory of our loved ones is as close to immortality as we can get.

The neurological peculiarity of Janet's illness killed the concept of "soul" that I was taught as a child. The disease reinforced to me that what the philosophers and theologians conceptualized as soul – simple, immaterial, intangible, yet giving us the capacity for reason, judgment, movement and will – were really just compartmentalized functions of our brains. Yet, with a little help from Vodou and the pelicans, I could see Janet has a soul again, and a shot at immortality, thanks to the good life she led - to her devotion to our family and to teaching and the example she set in the face of unimaginable suffering. Life and death were inextricably intertwined – the process of evolution refining and perfecting, slowly but inexorably evolving our spirit, our souls. We should accept death, therefore as the price we pay for the evolution of spirit.

We had met Baron Samedi at the crossroads of life and death, past and future. My path was now clear. Janet and I had formed a biologic and social union, the sum of which was greater than the individual parts. She brought our children into the world. We had raised them together. There is survival value for some of us, at least, in mating for life. I would nurse her through the difficult days ahead, honoring my commitment "till death do us part." Her soul would live on after her death, kept alive by the memories of our family.

39
All Saints' Day

Janet enjoyed holidays, and Halloween was high on her list of favorites. Prior to her illness, for more than twenty years, she would don a witch's costume and "haunt" both the Cushman School and the annual Halloween party held in our neighborhood. She loved the ritual of costuming, opting for a customized witch look, with a third eye on her forehead, green skin and several large ersatz warts on her nose and chin.

This particular Halloween, however, Janet realized she didn't have the strength to participate in the neighborhood party. Nor did she have the stamina to apply layer upon layer of makeup by herself. Halloween would become the first milestone of things given up, as Janet walked her path through the crossroads. We talked about it as I helped her with her makeup, an elaborate application of green and white face paint, black lipstick and eye shadow, and those repulsive plastic warts. She just didn't have the strength to go to the party, she concluded with resignation. She still, however, had enough stamina to surprise one more class with her transformation from teacher to witch.

I never really understood Janet's fascination with Halloween. Nor, for that matter, did I understand the significance of the holiday – sending our children out dressed as witches, goblins and ghosts, all for a few pieces of candy. Somehow modern Halloween seemed a symptom of a culture gone wrong. I shared this unease with Judith, my administrator, the following day. Judith is Haitian-American. Judith had started the conversation by inquiring as to how Janet was doing. I responded by relating the bitter sweetness of assisting her in getting ready for what would surely be the last of a series of holidays for her.

"It's sad," I confided in Judith. "Her hands are slowly getting weaker. She's been celebrating this holiday for years. She really gets into it. It's clear that she won't be able to do this again. I have to tell you, though, I didn't do well with the makeup. It was bizarre, all this black and green paste, trying to make her look like a dead person. When she was healthy, the dead look was like a joke. This year, it's a little too close to home."

I grew more pensive as we talked.

"I mean, I suppose looking like death is okay when you're young and think you'll live forever and death is something you feel you can mock and get away with it. I never realized it before last night, but in our culture, we trivialize death, be it in traditions like Halloween, in the way we portray death in the movies, or with this Gothic phase all the kids nowadays seem to be going through."

Judith had come in to discuss our budget, but something I said must have struck a responsive chord.

"We have a totally different view of death in Haiti, you know," she said. "Our dead are always with us. Today is one of the biggest holy days in Haiti – All Saints Day – a day to remember ancestors and to leave offerings on their graves. Afterwards we gather together and tell stories of the departed. Sometimes we laugh, sometimes we cry, but we know they are there with us.

"You Americans are in denial about death," Judith continued. "For us Haitians, death is part of life."

"Yes, I know," I said, nodding. "You can see it in Haitian funerals. They start off with grieving and wailing and dirge music, but they end with a celebration of the dead person's life."

"Dr. Fournier, there's a story that's told in Haiti of a doctor who starts his daily rounds at the Port au Prince cemetery, spending a few moments to pay respect to his patients who've gone on before him. He observes that faithful ritual every day."

"That's beautiful, Judith – can you imagine anything like that ever happening here in the United States? Here, as soon as you're dead, your doctor forgets you. Sometimes, if your memory fails, if you end up in a nursing home, you're forgotten by your family even before you die. I like the Haitian way better. In fact, I think I'll start doing that daily – not going to the cemetery, but spending some time remembering my patients, my family, and my friends who've gone on before me."

"Well, tell Janet I'm praying for her," Judith continued. Somehow, talking about the budget just didn't seem right at the moment.

"That's very sweet Judith. I have to tell you, though, prayers don't seem to be working. You're praying, my mom's praying, along with her sisters, Larry Pierre has got all of Little Haiti praying, the entire Commune of Thomonde is praying. The prayers don't seem to be working."

"Prayers always work, Dr. Fournier," Judith continued with a knowing smile. "You just have to know the right things to ask for. You don't always know how God answers, and you might not like what He says, but He always does."

The budget matters Judith needed to discuss were straightforward, and after she left I had time to reflect upon our conversation. Perhaps I was wrong to criticize my culture's trivialization of death – mocking death or trivializing it helps us cope with the bleak certainty of our mortality. As long as it wasn't carried to extremes, it was probably a good thing. But the Haitian way seemed clearly better to me. It offered a simple path to immortality – live well and you'll be remembered well by your family and your community. For a long time I had thought a lot about my dead patients, particularly my Haitian patients: Regis the dentist and all the others who died in the early days of the AIDS epidemic haunt me to this day. I thought often about my own family members who had died, particularly my grandparents, who I realize now, I worshipped. If I couldn't physically visit the graves of my patients, I could visit them in my mind daily. It was a tradition I would start that day, fittingly, All Saints Day.

The *Lwa*, the Vodou saints, represent a pantheon of all living things, for all life is animated by Spirit. There are eternal Lwa responsible for intercession in specific human abstractions – *Erzili Maron* for love, *Erzili Freda* for wisdom, *Damballah* for health, *Ogun* for victory over one's enemies. *Vodou*, however, also provides everyone an opportunity for sainthood. Everyone who lives the life of a Vodouisant becomes a Lwa after death – the reward for living a good life is eternal engagement with one's family. In a schema similar to Mahayana Buddhism or my grandmother's Italian - Catholicism, the *Vodouisants* have a panoply of spirits to advise, intercede and assist themselves and their progeny – a sharp theological contrast to orthodox Christianity, where sainthood is reserved for the exceptionally ascetic or pious.

Two holy days back to back in the liturgical calendar – All Souls Day followed by All Saints Day. In the western Catholic tradition, All Souls Day is for most of us mortals, those with enough unconfessed sins to deny us heaven on the first pass. In English-speaking countries, that holy day, intended to remind us of our mortality and exhort us to a righteous life, has morphed into Halloween, where the dead are mocked, children beg for candy, and parents worry about their safety. All Saints Day, reserved for the few souls who've been officially canonized, has taken backstage to the night of costumes and candy. In Haiti, there's no equivalent to Halloween, probably because there's no equivalent in Vodou to

Purgatory. Everyone aspires to sainthood, and almost everyone can achieve it. Yes, the Haitian way was better. I resolved to be Haitian in that regard – to remember my ancestors daily and to use holidays to tell stories about them to my children and (hopefully) grandchildren. Not just my ancestors though… Janet also would be in these stories. That's probably been Samedi's big joke all along – Janet the immortal. Janet the secular Jew becomes Janet the *Lwa*.

40
Entropy

I stared intently out the window, peering through the considerable overcast as the plane passed over Cite Soleil, just prior to landing. The ten months since I had last visited seemed far longer than it actually was, thanks to the daily drama of Janet's evolving illness. It had been almost a full year since she first started having symptoms and six months since she started to become progressively more dependent on me. Yet, there was no knowing how long it would take for her illness to play out. During that time, it was like I had a parallel life, wondering and worrying about my friends and patients back in Haiti while honoring my promise to stay with Janet while she was ill.

Then she had released me from that promise for four days. Everyone, including Janet, agreed; I needed a little time away, and had earned it. It was better that I go now – Suzanne, on winter break could stay with Janet while I was away. Janet's dependency on me and hence my responsibilities to be with her would surely increase as her illness progressed.

As I looked down on the rusted tin roofs, scattered like a tossed deck of cards, muddy waters covering the alleyways, schoolyard playgrounds and soccer fields reflected the shadow of our plane hurtling towards the runway. "A rare December deluge," I guessed. "It's supposed to be the dry season."

From the air, Cite Soleil looked as it had on a hundred and four previous passes. I wondered if it could really be as bad down there as the stories in The Herald portrayed it – daily murders, reports of corpses found in the first morning light, school children tiptoeing around still bleeding cadavers on their way to school – lives that could have been saved had there been an ambulance that worked and a driver not paralyzed by fear that he might be the next victim. Daily skirmishes by rival gangs, between gangs and police, and between *chimeres* and UN peacekeepers. Most of the victims were innocent bystanders. If these reports were true, it was a radically changed Cite Soleil from the slum that instilled me with such an odd sense of peace when I first visited it twelve years before.

Entropy run amok, I mused. Entropy – a truth so profound that one of its early discoverers, Ernst Boltzman, ordered its formula ($S = k \log W$) emblazoned on his tombstone, then committed suicide. It's the principle of thermodynamics that says that all energy systems, organic and inorganic, physical, chemical, and biologic, naturally tend to randomness and disorder. No matter how much energy you put into something to organize it, some of that energy must be dissipated as unproductive heat. In theory, the best you could do is break even. In practice, you could only lose.

As humans, we fear time, for we know the clock is ticking down on our mortality. But absent entropy, time is merely the measure of the relationship between distance and velocity. It's entropy that actually kills us. Bio-chemical entropy was killing Janet's neurons and sociopolitical entropy was killing Haiti. There didn't seem to be much I could do about either, no matter how much energy I expended. These musings ended abruptly as the plane's tires skidded onto the runway. The passengers broke into applause as the pilot braked and decelerated. I was back.

Suzanne's winter break did not overlap with my school's. That meant I wouldn't have students with me and, as I only had four days, I wouldn't have time to go to Thomonde. My mission, therefore, was focused on two groups of children in Port au Prince – Pere Luc's orphans at Bercail Bon Berger and children with hydrocephalus who had been shunted by one of Medishare's neurosurgeons two months before.

I was pleasantly surprised that renovations at the airport terminal had been completed - I passed through customs quickly, in air-conditioned splendor. I had only a small carry-on bag and my driver was waiting for me as soon as I stepped out the terminal's doors. Skilled in avoiding the roads notorious for kidnappings, he wove a new route up the back streets of Delmas towards Pétionville and the hotel where I would be staying - Villa Creole. The scenes unfolding before my window as we ascended – market women on the sidewalks with their eggplants and mangoes stacked in neat pyramids,; adolescent boys and girls in their school uniforms flirting with one another on street corners; wiry men pushing burettes (giant wheelbarrows) carrying seemingly impossible loads of cement blocks at the same speed as the slowly moving traffic - reassured me. It was just as always in Delmas, with no hint of the violence reported daily in the paper. However, Delmas was a working-class neighborhood, which, in Haiti, with its extremes of wealth and poverty, is the equivalent of a middle class neighborhood in the United States. The violence, of course, was confined to the slums surrounding the port: Bel Aire, Cite Militaire, and Cite Soleil, all several kilometers away in distance and light-years in terms of stability.

In surprisingly short order, given our circuitous detours, we arrived at Villa Creole. Tucked safely down a cul-de-sac far off the main Pétionville road, Villa Creole was the one place in Port au Prince where I could expect the same safety and hospitality I experienced in rural Thomonde. It was an older hotel – a vestige of a kinder and gentler time in Haiti's history – with elegantly hand-carved mahogany doors and trimmings, marble floors and Haitian artwork everywhere. At the same time, there was something akin to an atmosphere of Rick's Café surrounding Villa Creole – a product of its clientele, its staff and its proprietor.

Throughout the lobby and patio there were always clusters of people whispering in conspiratorial tones – members of Haiti's elite huddling with foreign businessmen or ambassadors, missionaries praying with their Haitian converts, and Haitian supplicants lobbying representatives of USAID. The hotel staff scurried between these groups, always smiling, always serving, repositories of probably millions of overheard rumors and secrets, but first and foremost loyal to the owner, Monsieur Roger. After all, they were among the lucky few in all of Haiti to have well-paying jobs.

They welcomed me each visit as if I were both long-lost family and returning war hero. Everyone from the porters through the front desk clerks to the maids and the waiters greeted me with that impeccable Haitian politeness married to that irrepressible Haitian smile. "Bienvini, Docté Fournier," each would say, in their turn, as I entered, registered, and was escorted to the best room in the hotel. It was a tradition Monsieur Roger insisted upon, in recognition of all Medishare was doing for Haiti. This visit, however, the staff's usual enthusiasm for my return was tempered by concern for Janet. Word had spread among them that she was ill.

"Y madame?" each would inquire. "Nou prie pou li!" ("And your wife? We're praying for her!")

"Prie pi fort!" I responded. "Li ampil malad!" ("Pray harder! She's very sick!")

I unpacked my bags and took a quick shower to wash off the diesel soot I had acquired on the ride up from the airport, and then went out to the pool patio for dinner. Roger, the owner, was there, talking intently with someone I didn't know. After a few minutes, however, he excused himself and joined me.

"Filbert – yon ver vin wouj pou dokte-la," he said just forcefully enough to be heard by the always attentive waiter, Filbert. Less than a minute later, a glass of red wine was delivered. "On me," said Roger with a broad smile. "It's been too long."

"Yes," I agreed. "Way too long."

I had last seen Roger in Miami, almost a year before, just before his wife died. Not wishing to open with really serious matters, I inquired about business. "The place seems busier than ever. I would have thought with all the bad press Haiti's been getting, you'd be deserted."

"Actually, business is booming," he said. "It's always good when the U.N.'s in town and there's no sign that they'll be leaving anytime soon. Plus, the interim government is bringing in all these consultants for security and the press corps is here - supposedly to cover the elections, although, trust me, they're not going to happen. But let's talk of more important things. How is Janet?"

"No, I'm not going to burden you with my troubles until first you tell me, how are you?"

"I'm moving on, Art. It's what Ariel wanted. I've thrown myself into my work and, you've probably heard, I'm dating someone. We'll probably get married. Ariel wanted that for me also."

Roger grew up in Patterson, New Jersey. He married Ariel, the girl next door, who just happened to be Haitian. Her father had built the hotel, and then fled to the United States during the Duvalier era. After the younger Duvalier fled Haiti for the south of France, Roger and Ariel returned to manage the hotel. Several years ago, Ariel was diagnosed with a slow-growing but incurable cancer. Single-minded in his devotion to his childhood sweetheart, Roger cared for his wife constantly as she developed one miserable complication of cancer after another. I saw her frequently at the hotel on many a prior visit and noted her determined dignity despite her decline. As Janet's illness evolved, I thought of Roger's and Ariel's ordeal often. His devotion served as an example to me, I told him.

"I find myself in a boat similar to the one you were in," I said of Janet. "Except the neurologists have even less to offer than the oncologists."

"Don't be so sure," Roger answered pensively. "That whole chemotherapy thing was way overrated. If I had to do it over again, I probably would have advised Ariel to quit after the third round. Those poisons just made her feel bad and the cancer kept spreading. But it's very hard to say no going into it when the doctors say there's some small chance it might help. At any rate, you're doing the right thing, being there for Janet. When it's all over with, you don't want to have any regrets. That will make it easier to move on, Art, and trust me, you have to move on."

After a bit more mutual commiseration, the conversation turned to Haiti. Roger was the best source of intelligence, in the military sense, about Haiti that I knew. The circumstances surrounding Aristide's departure, coupled with the attempts by the interim government to criminalize all of Aristide's political associates had only served to heighten the historic tensions between rich and poor. The UN had walled off the bastions of Aristide support, but, not wanting to risk casualties, failed to disarm neither the rebels who precipitated Aristide's departure nor his supporters. The slums of the capital had therefore become lawless free-fire zones. "You should talk to Father Rick before you leave, Art. He goes into Cite Soleil every day, trying to rescue the wounded."

"What about the countryside?" I inquired. "Any word from Thomonde?"

"As far as I know, things are quiet. Both Marie and Delva called earlier to make sure you got in safely. Marie's coming tomorrow night and Delva Friday morning. They'll be able to give you the whole story."

Roger then drew me into an in-depth discussion of the latest round of kidnappings. Some seemed purely criminal, others clearly had an element of political motivation. Political kidnappings were linked to both the left and the right, he explained.

The next morning I set out early for Bercail Bon Berger, the orphanage founded by Pere Luc, a priest I had searched for so diligently on Medishare's first visit. Medishare had been providing physical exams to his children since its early years and also screened them for tuberculosis – a serious problem in an orphanage where more than two hundred children slept in one large dormitory. My job for this visit was to follow up on the TB problem and also to check on the progress of one particular child, Dorsaintvil, whom we had brought to Miami for open heart surgery a year before. He had been complaining of chest pain, and Pe Luc was concerned his problem might have come back.

Bercail Bon Berger was built on several levels on the side of the same massive hill upon whose crest was the town of Pétionville. I entered through the back way so as not to have to fight my way through the throngs surrounding the street vendors who squatted in front of the main entrance on Delmas 48. To my surprise, the gate was locked. I rapped on the metal door and soon a child peered through a slit in the metal. After I introduced myself he ran away to fetch a security guard, complete with a shotgun slung over his shoulder, who let me in. "That's a new wrinkle", I thought. Security had never been an issue at the orphanage before.

I descended down through the complex, escorted by the security guard and the sentinel-child, looking for Pe Luc – past the library, rectory and dining hall down the path between the dormitory and playground, finally finding him in a little one-room study above the chapel. It was his hideaway - a place of relative quiet where he could escape for a few minutes at a time from the demands of hundreds of needy children. With the exception of the rectory and the study, children – mostly boys, although there were now, for the first time, some neighborhood girls allowed in during the day to attend the recently completed school. The school changed the whole atmosphere of the orphanage, with the organized recitation of lessons and singing of hymns drowning out the cacophony of the playground.

Luc and I embraced, after which he castigated me for being away so long. He was embarrassed when I explained that the reason was my wife's illness, and he promised to include her in his daily prayers. I inquired about Luc's own health – he was getting up there in years and had always complained of a persistent cough. "You've got to take care of yourself," I admonished. "All these kids depend on you. How many children do you have now?"

"It's getting close to three hundred now," said Luc with a wry smile, "not to mention the seventy five or so out at the farm in Leogane. Orphans are a growth industry here in Haiti. These days several new ones arrive at my door every week, wandering up from Cite Soleil and Bel Aire or carried up by the Sisters of Mercy."

"Well, I'll see the new ones who've arrived since my last visit…" I offered.

"Please do, and also, please check on Dorsaintvil – I always worry about him – he gets chest pains while running around the playground."

"No problem, Luc. Listen, what's up with the security guard?" I asked as I started to leave the study and begin my day's work. "Who'd want to kidnap these orphans?" I quipped.

Luc's visage transformed from smiling countenance to a pain-filled frown. "It's not them that's the target, it's me. I get money from wealthy Americans… Imagine that things have sunk that low. In all my years here, in all the bad times, no one, before now, would have ever thought of holding an orphanage priest for ransom!"

I embraced Luc again, and then went down to see the children awaiting me on the chapel steps below. For the next several hours it was like old times, just me and the children – half terrified, half fascinated by the prospect of being examined. Dorsaintvil turned out to be fine – just a little incisional tenderness. He had grown considerably since his surgery in Miami, recovering fully from the failure to thrive that resulted from the hole in his heart. The other children had a variety of minor conditions, most of which I could treat on the spot with the small stock of medicines in the dispensary. I joked with the children while I examined them and asked them about school, saving the painful parts – the vaccinations and skin tests for tuberculosis – for the very end.

The following day was equally rewarding. Treating children with hydrocephalus (children with giant heads) in-country was a first for Haiti, a small miracle Medishare had pulled off two months before, in spite of the political chaos and violence. It was important, however, to follow up on these kids, to make sure the shunting device, intended to return excess fluid from the brain to the abdominal cavity, had the desired effect. I marveled at the love given by the children's mothers and the missionary nurses caring for them, in spite of these children's persistent carnival side-show grotesqueness. The third day I returned to Bercail Bon Berger to "read" the skin tests for tuberculosis. Through constant surveillance of the new children and repeat testing of the old, we had cut the incidence of tuberculosis exposure in half.

"It was good to be back in Haiti, making a difference," I thought, as my plane back to Miami rolled down the runway. Given what I had accomplished in four short days, I should have felt better than I did – usually, returning home from Haiti, I'm positively exhilarated. Disquieting things had occurred on this trip, however. A conversation with Father Rick, the doctor-priest who had worked the streets of Cite Soleil daily, ministering to the dead and wounded, confirmed in graphic detail what I had gleaned from earlier conversations with Roger and Luc –Violence and kidnappings were real threats, not just exaggerations concocted by the media.

For twelve years I had injected enormous personal energy into Haiti, weaving an intricate tapestry of interwoven community health projects and training programs for Haitian doctors. In the ten months I had been away, our marvelous tapestry risked unraveling, just as Port au Prince had unraveled in chaos and disorder.

"Entropy!" I thought as the plane lifted skyward. "Entropy is killing us…"

41
Seizeman

> Meet me in the shadows
> Of some rainy morning,
> When the day is dawning
> And there's nothing you can do,
> I will comfort you...

As Janet's decline accelerated in the early months of 2006, this verse, from a song written by a college friend Dan, haunted me. The rest of the song was entirely forgettable college freshman angst – something about whiskey and roses and overdoses – but that first stanza's melancholy matched my mood. Janet was becoming increasingly debilitated by her disease. She was determined to continue teaching, in spite of the fact that I had to drive her to school and she needed a walker to steady herself as she stood or walked around the classroom. In addition to her weakness, she had developed a nagging cough, and, most troubling, shortness of breath when lying down. The cough signified the muscles of her throat were now involved – she was choking on her own saliva. More worrisome, her shortness of breath meant her diaphragm was also affected.

Janet refused to give in. She minimized her symptoms when she interacted with others – attributing her cough to allergies and her shortness of breath while lying flat to having old, worn-out pillows. At every stage of her illness she pushed herself beyond her physical limits, refusing to accept each new complication or limitation caused by her disease. She insisted she could still drive and frequently demanded the keys to her car, in spite of the fact that her hands were too clumsy and weak to turn the key in the ignition or to shift the transmission. She even let her second-graders take turns playing with her walker, pretending it was a miniature set of monkey bars. In reality, of course there were limits to what her will could accomplish. Each day the biblical passage "The spirit is willing but the flesh is weak" took new meaning, with greater poignancy.

It was touching to see her put up a bold front for her students every day, smiling and greeting the early arrivers as we entered. The love and respect her students gave her, which I had always known about in abstract terms, became palpably real to me. Even more touching was to see the creative ways by which she kept on teaching – first leaning against the wall rather than standing and later, when she was unable to stand, arranging her students' desks in concentric circles, with her sitting in the center. As one part of her nervous system rotted away, others blossomed to new heights, showing a strength of will, creativity, love, and passion for life I had previously taken for granted. She was losing her animus but growing in spirit. Janet, who had never before faced major adversity, was, in her own way, becoming a Vodouisant.

One day as I was helping her into her classroom, her walker caught in an imperceptible crack in the sidewalk - down she fell – it was impossible for me to catch her. Children and parents gathered around but she waved them off, simultaneously laughing and crying, saying "Well, that was silly," and then "its okay, I'm alright," in spite of obvious bruises and abrasions on her shins and elbows. As I picked her up – she was already too weak to stand up on her own – she whispered "We're going to have to come in earlier, before any of the children arrive."

I escorted her to her classroom, dusted off the dirt from her clothes, and cleansed her abrasions. I kissed her good-bye and pretended to leave then, instead, taking a circuitous route to the principal's office.

"How's Janet?" Cheryl, the principal, inquired. Word of her fall had evidently preceded me.

"She'll be okay," I responded. "Just a couple of scrapes and bruises. She's more embarrassed than anything."

"Cheryl, this is a battle we're not going to win…"

"Isn't there anything the doctors can do?" she said. "She's revered here, you know, our master teacher… We want to keep her going as long as we can – we'll do anything for her."

"That's very sweet, Cheryl. Her doctor is giving her medicines to ease the stiffness and her discomfort, but there's nothing they can do to stem the progression of her disease itself. You've seen how much worse she's gotten since the school year started…"

"I'd like you to think about how we could create a legacy for her here at the school," I went on. "Something really creative that will keep her memory alive as long as the school continues. I mean, I could build a hospital or clinic in Haiti and name it after her, but she never got into Haiti like I did. She loves Cushman, and she's loved teaching here."

I suggested we put together a committee of grateful parents, rattling of the names wealthy parents - potential donors-who knew her work.

I had come up with the idea of creating a legacy for Janet a few nights before. Janet's restiveness at night awoke me often. She needed me to reposition her, stretch her limbs, and re-stack her pillows under her head. She was also awakened by her dreams - "reverse nightmares" she called them, during which she was healthy and whole again. The nightmare began when she awoke and the dream ended. Once awakened, I could hardly ever get right back to sleep, a habit resulting from too many midnight awakenings during my internship. So, after she fell back asleep, I found myself, almost nightly, slipping out of bed, going downstairs, trying to make sense of it all. What possible meaning could there be in this curse of a disease inflicted on my wife – this cruel trick of Baron Samedi?

I tried distracting myself, to no avail, by channel surfing through the vapidity of late-night TV. I turned off the television and sat in the darkness. *M'pa dormi byen.* I'm not sleeping well. My soul is not at peace. The reason for my soul's disquiet was obvious – it was Janet's suffering and my impotence in the face of it. Here in America, insomnia is considered a medical illness, treated with pills. In Haiti, troubled sleep is seen as a malady of the spirit. If you live well – that is, following the *Vodouisant* way – working hard, giving love and respect to your neighbors and ancestors, the *Lwa* and to all you encounter, you'll sleep well. Untroubled sleep is, in effect, a gift from the *Lwa* for a well-led life.

Conversely, if you don't sleep well, you must be guilty of some moral transgression. Your sleep experience is a preview of your after-death experience – troubled sleep in this life portends anguish in the afterlife. Now, one might scoff at this as a simplistic worldview but the genius of *Vodou* is that is simple, rooted to the realities of life.

In *Vodou*, however, misfortune is not just a test of faith, but may also be seen as a cosmic punishment. There are two kinds of these cosmic punishments - a *huanga*, or curse inflicted by a priest, friend, or neighbor, or a *seizeman*, inflicted directly by the *Lwa*. In Janet's case, it was hard to believe this was a huanga, as she had ever violated society's norms or offended anyone. In fact, she was constantly concerned about what others might think and never committed so much as a traffic violation. Neither had she ever done anything to deserve a seizeman.

A *seizeman* is a paralysis, usually acute, but also possibly chronic. Where westerners would see a disease – a stroke, or Janet's case, ALS,

Vodouisants see an affliction imposed by the *Lwa*. A seizeman requires no human intermediary such as a *bokor* (Vodou priest) or *houngan* (spell-giver). Sitting in the darkness, I had to ask myself, what possible good could a benevolent spirit hope for by inflicting a curse on someone as horrible as ALS? Perhaps, it was so those who knew her would tell her story of heroism. Perhaps it was so we would create her a legacy.

Vodouisants create their legacy in four ways – through their art, through their children, through the communal memory of their goodness, and through their tombs. Haitians, like their West African cousins, believe that God the Creator is like an artist, creating something out of nothing. To be an artist is therefore to be like God. The Haitians, therefore, are a nation of artists, ranging from internationally renowned painters, to the cab driver that decorates every inch of his cab, and the child that makes marvelous kites out of plastic bags and twigs or toy trucks from cans and bottle caps. Many of these creations endure long after their creator has departed.

Children are raised to revere their parents and grandparents. Stories are told and passed on as part of the communal memory. Tombs are elaborate, aboveground affairs – often more elaborate than their occupant's house. If you ask a *Vodouisant* why they are building such an ornate crypt they will tell you "I live in my house just during my lifetime, but my tomb will be my home for eternity." All these aspects of Haitian culture are inextricably intertwined in the Vodou concept of respecting, revering, and keeping alive the memories of the dead.

In Janet's case, an elaborate tomb as her legacy was out of the question – she wanted to be cremated, and besides, she would consider it a waste of money. While I could count on our daughters to pass on stories of her, it was not necessarily a given that they would have children. So how would I create a legacy for Janet? Well, certainly we could do something at her school – the parents, teachers, and students were her community and it would be relatively easy to create a perpetuating communal memory there. She had turned teaching into an art form. I could work with the school to permanently institutionalize that memory.

I hummed the first verse of Dan's song to myself.

I will comfort you…" I thought, with the certainty that you'll always be remembered, venerated, and revered just as the Haitians had taught me. I'll make up for the years I took you for granted, and tell your story. Then, when it's over, perhaps I'll be able to sleep again.

Just then, Janet called me to re-arrange her pillows.

"Dying is greatly overrated," she quipped as I re-entered the bedroom. "Where were you?"

"Downstairs…"

"What were you doing?"

"Thinking…"

"Well?"

"I'm going to create a legacy for you. Your spirit is going to live forever", I whispered as I lifted her with one hand and propped three pillows behind her back with the other.

"Right. I'll believe it when I see it. Go to sleep, will you?"

42
Samedi's Revenge

Each day, between my trip to Haiti in December and Suzanne's graduation from dental school in June, heightened my anxiety and ambivalence. Janet so wanted to make it to this event in Anne Arbor, Michigan, and I was rooting for her to make it. There was no end, however, to the accumulation of her misery.

It was one thing to know what was going to happen to Janet in the abstract – the list of complications that had been ticked off by her neurologists – and another to live through them with her. Each day it seemed something worsened or weakened and she was forced to give up yet another fragment of her independence, dignity and privacy, the details of which are best left unsaid.

And yet, Suzanne's graduation turned out to be a truly joyous event. Janet beamed throughout the ceremony and afterwards, even though we had to prop her up against walls for the prerequisite family photos. Although Adrienne, my mother, sister and Janet's sister all made the pilgrimage to Ann Arbor, the major responsibility for Janet's care fell on my shoulders. It was a sobering prospect. I had to walk her everywhere, dress her, and take her to the bathroom. For months, her purpose in life had been making it to Suzanne's graduation. Once we got back to Miami, what would keep her going?

My feeling that Samedi had singled out Janet as revenge for the lives Medishare had saved in Thomonde gained credence when Marie forwarded me the report of the first three years of the Green Family Foundation Initiative – the grant that funded our community health worker project in Thomonde. The death rate there had dropped over 40 percent, resulting in at least five hundred lives saved in Thomonde alone, not counting the lives saved in Casse and Marmont, two communities adjacent to Thomonde that the Ministry of Health had assigned to Medishare in the second year of the Initiative. All told, Medishare was now responsible for the health care of 75,000 souls. No wonder Samedi was angry!

Janet asked if I would take her to Cape Cod one last time. Her brother had a lovely home in Yarmouthport, with a sweeping view of Cape Cod Bay and a first-floor guestroom so that we wouldn't have to go up and down stairs. It was her dying wish, and I knew it. To my surprise, however, seemingly out of the blue, she encouraged me first to go to Haiti for a few days, before we headed to Massachusetts. Suzanne would be home for four day before starting her residency program in pediatric dentistry. Suzanne would take care of her.

It was a sweet gesture on Janet's part. Haiti had been such a flashpoint in our lives. This was tacit acknowledgment on her part of how important my work there was to me – an act of reconciliation, and a reward for taking such good care of her in Ann Arbor. Medishare's June trip had already been scheduled for that week, so I could easily tag along, even on short notice. No matter that I'd have to leave Haiti a day early to make our flight to Boston.

The four days in Haiti were exactly what I had hoped for: intense, rewarding work, bonding experiences with our medical students and Haitian staff, coupled with the evenings' camaraderie, nurtured by the cuisine, libations, and entertainment provided by our Thomondois hosts – a way to re-charge my batteries in anticipation of what lay ahead.

Janet lived much longer than I ever thought possible. I really didn't expect her to last long after Suzanne's graduation, although I wasn't sure what would take her. When highly publicized cases of barely living patients such as Karen Quinlan or Terri Schiavo had surfaced in the media, Janet had always said "If I'm ever in that situation I'd want you to shoot me." She believed, in theory at least, in euthanasia. At one point, early in her disease, she even joked about moving to Oregon, the only state in which euthanasia is legal. Now she had morphine and sleeping pills – all the medicine she might need – yet she chose to endure an ordeal worse than Quinlan's or Schiavo's. She was slowly, relentlessly losing her voice and the use of her arms and legs. She was choking, coughing, and drooling a little more with each passing day. I'm not sure why she didn't choose the morphine option – perhaps it was the gradualness of her decline that made each new indignity bearable. Perhaps, in her mind, she traded the one big event that had kept her going (Suzanne's graduation) for a series of smaller events, like visits from family or the nightly phone calls from our daughters. Perhaps, thanks to her caregivers, she simply reached a mundane accommodation with a life of paralysis or a stoic acceptance of the fact that the unique experience of life itself was worth it, even if it had to be experienced by a mind entombed in a useless body. If the truth be known, however, I don't think any of these reasons explained her choice.

It takes courage to kill oneself, but it takes more courage to endure a disease as outrageously awful as Lou Gehrig's disease. Just as Christ, if the theologians are to be believed, willed to live through his passion to set an example of courage for his apostles, I think Janet willed to live through her own passion, in part, to set an example for our daughters.

A big part of what kept Janet going was the intensity of her love for our daughters and her desire to see them or talk to them yet one more time. As her illness progressed towards complete paralysis, Adrienne and Suzanne resolved that one or the other would visit every weekend. Bhudda taught that desire was the source of all suffering. In Janet's case, he was very close to the mark. To satisfy her desire to share one more minute with our daughters on weekends, she would endure five weekdays of doing nothing except letting others attend to her bodily functions. But Bhudda was wrong in saying that the way to end the suffering was to end desire. Desire to live and to have a few moments with our daughters, family, and friends made the endurance of her ordeal, for Janet at least, worth it. Suffering was the crucible that brought forth her spirit.

I wish I could tell you that the closeness that reemerged in our relationship early on in Janet's illness persisted until the very end, but I would be lying. We had two good years, but in the end, entropy and Samedi conspired to frustrate us. Elizabeth Kubler-Ross, among the wisest writers about death, formulated that dying patients pass through stages of anger, denial, bargaining, and finally acceptance. In Janet's case, at least, acceptance came early, followed by regression to anger and denial. A lot of that anger spilled over to me. As it became clearer and clearer that I would outlive her, Janet became obsessed with what my life would be without her. Her reasoning powers were frequently clouded by morphine and valium. She was convinced at one point that I was trying to drive her to suicide, so I could get on with my life. The more dependent on me she became, the less she was willing to admit how much she needed me. She also had times when she believed that her caregivers were also trying to kill her. In retrospect, it was a full-blown case of paranoia, probably caused by too much morphine.

Her last weeks were a crescendo of frustration for me and for her, as her voice relentlessly eroded from difficult to impossible to understand. The end-stages of Lou Gehrig's disease are torture for both its victims and their loved ones. Those frustrations, in turn, challenged my commitment to do the right thing. Hours passed attempting to interpret her slurs, grunts and groans. My life was on hold. I had the means, in the form of morphine, sleeping pills, and sedatives to end Janet's suffering at will. In the final analysis, however, euthanasia for my convenience and not by her choice would have been murder, no matter how I rationalized it. So I endured her frustrations with her, until her final moments arrived.

Two weeks before she died, the development of bedsores, her unintelligible speech, the inability to chew and swallow and worsening problems breathing forced her to the decision that she "wanted out" – a decision she shared with me and her hospice doctor during one of his home visits. That day she accepted the fact that she could no longer swallow without choking – for two weeks before she had survived only on ice tea, ice cream and mashed potatoes. She asked the doctor only that she have enough pain medicine to sedate her until she lapsed into a coma.

Adrienne, Suzanne, my sister Mary and I kept the final vigil. Denise, one of her faithful attendants, offering her drops of apricot nectar laced with methadone, her medicine for pain, to assuage her thirst. Stopping eating and drinking is supposed to lead fairly quickly to dehydration, followed a few days later by a peaceful death in one's sleep. Experts in thanatology (the study of death) claim it is the preferred method of dying for the hopelessly ill. So much for theory, at least in Janet's case. We kept up a small amount of fluids for two days to allow her family to fly in from Boston for one last visit. She practiced smiling for their arrival and held up well for most of their visit, dissolving into tears only at the end.

Shortly thereafter, however, she regained her composure. She asked to delay taking her methadone and sedative for a while and watched television with our daughters. At 11:00, she stoically took her medicine and slipped into a profound, prolonged sleep.

She slept for thirty-six hours and her pulse and respiratory rate dropped, giving me hope her death would be peaceful as planned. But a problem in hospice's weekend coverage and difficulties in swallowing a key pain medicine led to her awaking with severe chest pain, necessitating both morphine and methadone elixirs every two and three hours, respectively. The problem was she could not swallow correctly, so she aspirated each dose of medicine. Soon she had pneumonia, and with it a high fever, labored breathing and a deep blue discoloration of her nose, lips hands and feet – a result of a lack of oxygen. That blueness, coupled with the wasting caused by her disease and acute and chronic starvation made her appear like some bizarre skeletal Halloween ghoul, mocking her former beauty. Her doctor ordered morphine suppositories, but there were none in stock in South Florida, so she suffered with chest pains and pneumonia, semi-alert, for eighteen hours until a narcotic patch, ordered by the hospice doctor on call, arrived via courier at 1:30 a.m. Thanks to that patch, she slipped back into coma. It took another two days before her heart and lungs gave out.

Adrienne, Suzanne and I were with her when her chest stopped rising and falling. I pondered the joy of our young romance, the sometimes difficult times in the middle of our marriage, and the horrific details of her final ordeal. The marathon was over. I had kept my word to care for Janet at home, in spite of the difficulties of the last few weeks of her existence, when the combination of morphine, fatigue, hunger and despair took away those last aspects of her soul – her fighting spirit and her ability to laugh in the face of death – that her disease itself could not touch. No, the last few weeks had been hell for her and hell for me - she alternatively hallucinating, angry, delusional and frightened, me helpless as the final stages of her disease unfolded. I grieved then. Now was a time to move on. We were both at our Vodou crossroads – she from existence to memory, men spiritual drift to the life of a Vodouisant.

My daughters and I hugged and kissed her and then held each other. After a while we called my mother, her brother and her best friends to initiate a series of phone calls to get the word out. The end to her suffering had finally, mercifully arrived. Janet was cremated, as she wished. A week after her death, we celebrated her life in a memorial service at the Cushman School, where she taught for so many years. Over four hundred family, friends, and former students attended.

43
Postscript to One Disaster and Prelude to Another

Intellectually, I had prepared myself for Janet's passing, beginning as soon as I heard her diagnosis. With each day she lost strength, I had steeled myself in anticipation of her eventual passing. I even rationalized it as a blessing, given all she went through. Living through the aftermath, however, was another thing entirely. The relief I experienced when she died soon dissipated into grief, no matter how much I tried to intellectualize it away. Grief is a natural process, not to be denied. For the longest time, I didn't sleep well – afflicted with haunting dreams of Janet's suffering, a recurrent bizarre but strangely realistic dream that she was still alive, and the whole Lou Gehrig's thing never happened. On the outside I seemed OK to others. Spirit is a fragile thing, however, and wounds to the spirit take longer to heal than wounds to the flesh.

The lessons I'd learned from Haiti's people enabled me to not just endure but to understand. In Haiti wisdom is cultivated through parole *granmoun* – sayings passed down from generation to generation. For example, the title of Tracy Kidder's best-seller, "Mountains Beyond Mountains" is derived from the saying *"deye morn gin morn"* – "on the other side of the mountains, more mountains" – a perfect metaphor for the challenges of life in the impoverished country whose name means "land of mountains." For every *parole granmoun* that captures the hardships and challenges of Haitian life, however, there is an uplifting one. Perhaps the most beloved is, *Lespwa fe viv* – hope makes us live.

That said, for two and one-half years after Janet's death, I went through the motions at work. I took some solace in trips to Thomonde, our headquarters in the Central Plateau with my medical students. Barth, with the help of Michel and Marie, kept Project Medishare going through bad times.

In the power void and class struggles that erupted in 2005-2006, both sides of Haiti's polarized political spectrum supported gangs of paramilitary forces to achieve their political goals. Acquiring or keeping power in Haiti required patronage. Dispensing that patronage took priority over maintaining law and order. For couple of years, kidnappings and violence, once rare in the capital and unknown in the countryside, proliferated.

It was not until 2009 that the situation began to improve. President Preval proved more pragmatic, less doctrinaire, than Aristide. He was willing to work with the U.S. administration rather than provoke them. Former President Clinton brought engaged Haiti into his Clinton Global Initiative, promoting international aid, and a return of international assistance. The Obama Administration increased aid, and other international donors followed. Even Mother Nature cooperated – there were no major storms or flooding during the 2008 and 2009 rainy seasons, allowing foreign assistance in those years to go towards infrastructure development rather than disaster relief. The road up to Thomonde was finally paved, shortening our transit time from four to two and one/half hours.

It had been more than thirty years since I had met my first Haitian patients, suffering from what we now know to be AIDS. It had been fifteen years since, almost by chance, Project Medishare was first organized. In the past ten years, the three communities we worked within the Central Plateau had moved from no health care through episodic care provided by Medishare volunteers to continuing care provided by Haitian doctors, nurses and health workers. As a result, mortality in Thomonde and its surrounding communities plummeted. More importantly, we – Medishare volunteers and our Haitian colleagues – brought hope back to tens of thousands of people living on the central plateau.

"Yes, things were better," said everyone in Port au Prince. The clothing industry assembly shops were re-opening, paying workers there a whopping $4 a day. The capital now had electricity eight hours a day. Tourism was rebounding. Royal Caribbean Cruise Line built a huge dock to accommodate its passengers at its Haitian resort in Labadee, while American hotel chains vied with Haitian proprietors to accommodate the increased numbers of foreigners coming in and out of Port au Prince. Missionaries, who drastically curtailed activities during the bad times, returned in ever-larger numbers. By early 2010, there were an estimated 35,000 foreigners in the country, including 20,000 Americans.

These developments did little to address the root causes of Haiti's problems: the collapse of the rural economy in the decades prior to the earthquake, which forced peasants to move to the slums of the city, squatting on and building makeshift housing on land that was actually uninhabitable — steep mountain slopes, ravines and dry river beds. I had watched these bidonvilles for years, growing incessantly like a cancer, from the rooftop of the Hotel Villa Creole during my stays there. I was always concerned a storm or hurricane would wash them away. Never did I consider the possibility of an earthquake.

The days of ambivalence between Project Medishare and the school were over. We were one of the few organizations actually addressing the problems of rural Haiti head on. We had expanded from heath care to pilot projects in education and agriculture. Our responsibilities had also grown. We were employing about one hundred workers who cared for over 85,000 people. Donors in South Florida had given us enough money to build a maternity center for round-the-clock obstetrical care, a new, larger guesthouse, and an innovative nutrition program centering on the production of a nutritious porridge.

The problem was finding funds for continuing operations. Haiti had always been a "tough sell" to philanthropists, and crash of 2008 in the United States made fundraising for Haiti all the more difficult. Donor fatigue, compounded by the financial crisis of the U.S. economy, dried up our sources of money. Our expenses were three times our income. In December 2009 we faced the prospects of lay-offs and curtailment of services. Project Medishare was on the verge of bankruptcy.

And then, on January 12, as I was driving home from work, Baron Samedi played his biggest trick.

Part III
Lespwa Fe Viv

44
Total Save

Day six after the quake...

By the morning following her rescue, the resuscitation and evacution of the baby had become a global media phenomenon. Elizabe Cohen's story of the tiny infant pulled from the rubble was broadca constantly on CNN and other news outlets picked up on the story, n the least because it ended happily.

. Karen, the nurse, visited Jenny in the Pedi-ICU and phoned in a fo low-up report – the amount of bleeding under the skull fracture w minimal and only a small amount of supplemental oxygen was need to ease her breathing. Her kidneys were working remarkably well – ki ney failure is a big problem for patients in shock or with crush injuri The weakness on the right side of her face had totally resolved and s appeared developmentally normal for her suspected age. In other wor barring unforeseen complications, she should make a full recovery.

"A total save!" beamed Karen, the pediatrician, when she heard the report. "Yes!" she exclaimed, pumping her fist in a manner mimicking Alonzo's signature gesture. Her obvious pride in her accomplishment was certainly justified. It was extraordinary, really, not only for a pediatric resuscitation to be executed this flawlessly but also to result in a totally positive outcome.

Alonzo and Elizabeth Cohen of CNN wanted to be "de-briefed" in more detail about what happened when the plane arrived in the United States. When I had returned from the airport, however, Elizabeth had raised concerns about the State Department's ban on the evacuation of Haitians. Did taking Baby Jenny out of the country violate departmental policy? Pumped on adrenaline, I replied, "I don't care about the State Department!"

For Elizabeth, this was her job – just part of good reporting – another remarkable aspect of an extraordinary story. Alonzo had a more philosophical perspective. Product of a Jesuit education at Georgetown, he was outraged that there were laws or regulations that might have threatened the life of a child. Not just this child, but any child.

Later that evening, Alonzo took me aside. He promised he would do something for Medishare "in a big way."

"That baby and this whole experience has changed my life," he told me.

I knew the feeling.

45
Lost and Found

As soon as his home site came into view, Junior knew this day would be different. His neighbors were standing at the highest point of rubble, scanning the street he was ascending. It was the fifth day after the quake, and he was running a little later than usual. Nadine had improved to the point where she could now get out of the car and walk with his assistance. But each morning he had to bring her food, wash and dress her. He also needed to find a place they could stay, as they could not live in a parking lot forever.

When the neighbors spotted him, they gestured with their hands for him to come quickly. He started running and as soon as he was within earshot, they started yelling. "They found your baby! They found your baby!"

Junior was still too far away to decipher their countenances. Finding her didn't mean finding her alive. Even though he had returned every day, at Nadine's insistence, in his heart, hope was ebbing away. As he got closer, however, he could see they were smiling.

"Is she alive?"

"Yes!"

"Who found her?"

"*Blan!* They had dogs!"

"Where is she?"

"They took her to the hospital."

Junior hugged his neighbors, thanked them, and then sprinted down Canapé Vert to the neighborhood hospital – the same hospital to which he had carried Nadine. He stopped first at the car he left her in to share the news. She wept for a moment, praised God, then sent her husband to find her child. His first stop was the hospital itself. To his astonishment, the head nurse there had no knowledge of an infant being admitted.

Where could she be? Off he sped to the General Hospital – the public hospital near the presidential palace. It was partially damaged in the quake, but its emergency room was open and it was the traditional hospital for emergencies to be taken. The nurse there told him they had no infant brought in from Canapé Vert that day, but generously offered him to tour the unit. He diligently inspected every crib. No Jenny. At Hopital De La Paix – the other public hospital, closer to the airport – it was the same story. No Jenny.

Junior trudged back to Nadine's bedside – a journey on foot that took almost two hours.

"I could not find her," he reported.

Nadine embraced him. "It's alright. God has spared her. God will deliver her. Rest now. You'll find her tomorrow…"

46
Obsession

Upon returning home to Miami after my first earthquake "tour of duty," it was fascinating to watch how the media dealt with the evolving story in Haiti. Most stations were still giving twenty-four hour coverage and most newspapers gave at least one front page spread each day. There was, of course, a daily morbid fascination with the rising death toll and at least one "feel good" story per day like CNN's story of the infant plucked from the rubble. As each day passed, some reporters even "got it" that there was something special about the Haitian people. I started hearing praise of their resilience, toughness, and spirituality. It was a rare reporter, however, that could entirely shake off the legacies of prejudice and stereotype that comes with being an American.

By the second week after the quake, many reporters were expecting, even predicting riots, and looting. Small incidents, often provoked by relief agencies dropping food from helicopters, were magnified out of proportion. The conventional wisdom went something like this – surely, if an event of this magnitude had happened in a major city in the United States, there would be riots and looting. Look what happened after Katrina. When law and order are disrupted, poor folks turn to crime. Haiti was universally poor, so we should expect these behaviors to be rampant. With each passing day, we heard of "rising tensions," as food and water were painfully slow in coming. U.N. troops were ordered to shoot to kill suspected looters. Armed troops patrolled neighborhoods with guns at the ready. In reality, in spite of hunger, thirst and deprivation on an unprecedented scale, the people did not act out, they simply endured. Now, one might ask why authorities could not differentiate between breaking into a building and stealing merchandise and scavenging through rubble for survival. Children and youth were shot as a result of this confusion. All of which begs the larger question: why this obsession with rioting and looting?

The simple answer is, because Americans impose their experience on Haiti. If there is a breakdown of law and order in the United States, it not uncommon for violence to erupt because of unresolved tensions surrounding issues of race, as well as the persistent belief among minorities that the instruments of law and order are in actuality instruments of repression. In Haiti, hatred between the races dissipated after 1805, when all whites either left the country or were executed by order of President Dessalines. Tensions rose again during the U.S. occupation of 1915-30, particularly in the countryside. Today, however, the sighting of a "blan" in rural Haiti mostly evokes nothing more than curiosity.

In rural Haiti, where government is at best absent and at worst an instrument of repression of the majority, it is social relations that maintain order. The solidarity of common cause that arose in Haiti's revolution was reinforced by a West African way of life that, thanks to the historic isolation of Haiti in general and rural Haiti in particular – has yet to be polluted by global acculturation. One is expected to not commit crimes, but to help and support one's neighbor, particularly in hard times. One is expected to live the life of a Vodouisant – even after an earthquake.

Skeptics might argue that the earthquake struck the capital which is dominated by a culture created by an urban aristocracy. However, over the past four decades, the population of Port au Prince has swelled from half-million to two million people – almost all peasants emigrating from the countryside. The values of rural Haiti have proven durable and adaptable. They survived, largely intact, the hard times of the Duvaliers, the Generals, Aristide, and the interregnum of 2005-2006 when Aristide was forced from power. After the earthquake these values insured there would be little looting or violence. Those same values are the key not just to Haiti's survival but its resurrection.

47
Our Dead Will Always Be With Us

Vodouisants revere their ancestors. That reverence dictates a proper funeral and burial. In Port au Prince, before the earthquake, along the sidewalks bordering the General Hospital, coffin-makers proudly displayed their handiwork. Funeral directors ranked in status with physicians and lawyers. In the countryside, every small hamlet has a coffin-maker. In towns too small for a doctor or village priest, the funeral director is often the most prominent citizen. In deference to the acceleration of decay fostered by tropical heat, funerals usually happen shortly after death. Loved ones grieve openly and passionately in the beginning. When the brass band arrives (as incongruous as it sounds, every village has a brass band – some could rival New Orleans' best), first dirges, reflecting the sadness of the loss and then rhythmic celebrations of the departed's life and the fact that his or her spirit – *"ti bon ange,"* or "good little angel" is freed from the miseries of life and free to join the *"gwo bon ange"* - the collective spirit of Lwa.

Yet, a mystical connection forever exists between the *"ti bon ange"* and its *"corpse cadaver"* – its earthy remains. Tombs therefore become very important – elaborate above-ground tombs, with spires and crosses and a flat roof that forms a table for loved ones to leave offerings of food and rum on birthdays, anniversaries and the holiest days --All Saints Day on November 1 and Ancestors Day which occurs on New Year Day, January 1, which also happens to be Haitian Independence Day.

There's no coincidence in any of this. "Toussaint" (All Saints) is a common name in Haiti, reflecting the community of spirit of the collective Lwa. And just as the mythic god Janus looked both forward and backward, the *Vodouisant* on New Year's Day looks forward to the future and back to the past, celebrating both the living and the departed. New Years, then, is a celebration of the crossroads, that Vodou abstraction of the intersection of past, present and future, life, death and eternity.

In Haiti, even soup has spiritual significance. On New Years, families cook *"soup jimou"* – "pumpkin soup" and carry it to the homes of families and friends, sharing it almost as communion. The legend has it that during their ancestors' enslavement, only their masters were allowed the delicacy of soup jimou. So the soup is a symbol of their ancestors struggle and their birthright of freedom. Several of my Haitian friends brought me pumpkin soup on New Years after Janet died. Yes, our dead are always with us.

"Papa Doc" Duvalier, Haiti's infamous dictator from 1957 to 1971, knew this aspect of the national character well and used it as a psychological instrument of repression. There's an infamous spot on the road out of Port au Prince at the base of the coastal mountains, called *Titayen*. It's only a few miles from Port au Prince, but arguably the most desolate and austere landscape in the country- a desert-like moonscape where volcanic rocks are punctuated by an occasional cactus or thorn acacia.

Papa Doc's henchman would leave the bodies of their victims there, unburied, so that their eyes could be plucked out by crows and their flesh scavenged by goats and vultures before their families could find them. You can now drive from Port au Prince to *Titayen* in a matter of minutes, thanks to a new paved road, but the place is as desolate as ever and forever seared in infamy in the national psyche.

Everyone knows the story of the victims of *Titayen*, except the person, whoever it was, that chose it as the site of the mass graves for earthquake victims. That person, probably from the United Nations, was certainly not Haitian. No *Vodouisant* would treat the dead like that. In the first morning light after the quake, streets were littered with corpses. By evening that day, bodies that could be identified by their families were already carried away for burial. Those that couldn't were being moved to sidewalks, arranged in rows and covered by sheets. Crews of Haitians spontaneously organized themselves to excavate buildings by hand – not just to find survivors, but to recover the dead also. By post-quake day three, however, the international cleanup crews arrived. What to do with all the dead bodies became the issue of the day.

There were several issues, really. The difficulties of relief trucks navigating rubble-stricken streets were compounded by human remains that could not just be driven over. The sheer numbers involved, with estimates at that time climbing by tens of thousands daily, challenged those responsible for planning their removal. The biggest issue, however, was the hysteria over the alleged public health risks all these dead bodies represented.

In truth, the dangers of decomposition are greatly exaggerated. The diseases that often break out amidst disasters, such as cholera and dysentery, are the result of poor sanitation among the living, not the decay of dead people. Decay is part of the cycle of life. In fact, without decay, life would cease on earth. There are entire species – saprophytes and scavengers – that make their living out of corrupting or consuming our flesh. The problem is that death stinks. The stench of death hung over the entire city.

The clean-up teams, whose origins were unknown, decided that something needed to be done. In spite of the fact that survivors were anxiously still searching for loved ones, and that thousands of victims had already been found by their families and properly buried, the teams dug large pits in the middle of the night. Contorted bodies (rigor mortis had long set in, freezing the victim's bodies in their agonal positions) were scooped up by front-end loaders and hauled by dump trucks to the pits.   When discovered by the media a week later, most of the corpses were still fully or mostly exposed to the tropical sunlight and scavenging birds.   The cameras focused on exposed torsos and limbs and the reporters warned that the pictures might be too graphic for some.

What the cameras could not convey was the smell of death, now a hundred times worse than in the city. What they also didn't show was that, in spite of that stench, survivors had started to arrive, still hopeful they might find loved ones, stomaching the visceral horror and stench to search the pits for loved ones, and to gather with others before leaving to sing hymns and to pray.

48
Spiritual Orphans

My unhappiness with the media over their portrayal of Haiti's vulnerable children had been simmering even before the Idaho Missionary caper. So-called experts from international agencies flooded the airwaves with warnings of the danger of child trafficking created by the earthquake. The implication, both stated and unstated, was that these problems were the Haitians' fault - that there was something about the Haitian worldview, culture or "lifestyle" that enabled these abuses.   W h e n ten Baptist missionaries from Idaho were arrested for trying to transport thirty-three alleged Haitian "orphans" across the border with the Dominican Republic without proper documentation, my anger reached a proverbial boil.

These missionaries were initially portrayed as, at best, heroes, at worst, naïve but well-intentioned do-gooders. The Haitian government was the villain. As the possibility that the missionaries might be involved in some kind of human trafficking became more plausible (particularly when it was revealed that the missionaries were being advised by a lawyer wanted for child-prostitution in El Salvador), the storyline split, with some accounts emphasizing the innocence of all the missionaries, save the "ringleader," other focusing on the cynicism of Haitians who want to give up or sell their children. Was it realistic to expect the media to do some investigative reporting on the whole missionary phenomena?

Of course, there are missionaries have done a lot of good and who aspire to the noblest in human nature. But what is it about missionaries that make them assume that there are so many Haitians in need of salvation?

Haitians adore and revere their children for their innocence, just as they revere old people for their wisdom. The Kreyol word for child *'ti-moun"* is derived from the French "petit monde" – literally, the world of the little ones – giving them a status equal to the *"gwo-moun"* (adults) and *"gran moun"* (old/wise folks). Each child, no matter how poor, has a "Sunday best." For boys, it's a suit and tie, for girls, it's a frilly dress, accompanied with lace and ribbons. These traditions are rooted in West Africa, where to be adorned in finery is a mark of royalty. They are also reinforced by the collective memory of slavery, when masters were dressed in Paris fashions, and kept slaves naked.

Even in the best of times, however, many children are orphaned because life expectancy for Haitians is in the high forties or low fifties. Historically Most of these children were taken up by close relatives – grandparent, aunts, uncles, or older siblings and raised with the same love and respect as their newfound brothers and sisters. Problems arose, however, when families left their ancestral communities in the countryside, as a survival choice, and fled to the slums of the city, or sent their children to distant relatives or acquaintances because they could no longer feed them or send them to school. Children whose parents died in the slums of Haiti's cities became institutionalized orphans, while those sent to the city to be cared for by distant family or strangers came to be known as *"restaveks"* ("stay withs"). In the absence of a governmental safety net, the restavek phenomenon filled a void. It amounts to a barter system in which the host agrees to feed and clothe the restavek while sending them to school. In exchange, the restaveks perform household chores. Given the alternatives, for most restaveks, this was a fair bargain.

Not all *restaveks* were poor. Some were simply the illegitimate offspring of prominent scions. In a certain sense, some *restaveks* filled a role similar to house servants in colonial days – a notch above the life of a field slave. All servants, *restaveks* or not, are potential victims for abuse, if their situation is desperate enough and their masters that unscrupulous. Given the extremes of wealth and poverty in Haiti, it's surprising it doesn't happen more often. Orphans are also vulnerable – not just for physical abuse but spiritual abuse also – which brings us back to the missionaries from Idaho.

To many Protestant missionaries, Vodou is something akin to "black magic." Even those Protestant orphanages managed by Haitian pastors are usually supported by a U.S. church. The primary mission of these orphanages is not just to feed and clothe but save souls from *Vodou*. Yet, if you cut off a Haitian child from *Vodou*, you steal part of their identity, cutting them off from their roots in ancestral Africa; from Vodou's intense, Dionysian spirituality; from its search for meaning in everything from its reverence for young and old; from its communality with all other Vodouisants, living and dead who share this worldview. This explains why many Haitians viewed the motivation of these missionaries with suspicion and why the Haitian government was right to stop them at the border. For Haitians, Vodou is neither a black magic nor a religion. It is a way of life.

49
In-Tents-ive Care

True to his word, Alonzo Mourning returned to Miami after five days of service, having dedicated himself to Medishare "in a big way." Within a day of his return he had recruited several other athletes into an organization he named "Athletes Helping Haiti" which raised millions of dollars for our work. He cajoled his former team, the Miami Heat, into donating four large "event tents" that we could turn into our own field hospital, outside the U.N. compound.

In Haiti, Barth Green took the lead. He negotiated with the Haitian Government for the use of a large tract of land at the end of the airport runway. The tents arrived just a week after the earthquake. They were set up in four days. Ten days after the quake, we successfully transferred three hundred patients out of the U.N. tents, into our new home. The following day, President Rene Preval dedicated the hospital.

The move came none too soon. Our hospital census had been growing daily, as patients were continuously brought in, but had no homes to go home to. Without running water, toilets, or air conditioning, sanitation was abysmal. The stench of urine, feces, sweat and pus inside the tents co-mingled with the smell of death wafting in from whatever breeze managed to find its way into the compound. We had about one hundred new volunteers arriving daily but no place to eat or sleep. Given the un-sterile conditions and close quarters, the number of post-op infections was rising dramatically.

Donors large and small from around the world gave equipment, supplies, medicines, and their own time to support our effort. Within days of it opening, the field hospital had two functioning operating rooms, anesthesia machines, an x-ray unit, an ICU with monitors and four respirators, and a well-stocked pharmacy. Donations of satellite phones, computers and good-old-fashioned ham radios allowed us to set up a communication center in the field hospital and a "command center" at our medical school. Daily briefings occurred and methods for instantaneous problem-solving rapidly evolved. For instance, when a case of suspected diphtheria was brought in, we shipped out diphtheria antitoxin the following morning.

Admittedly, running a field hospital in circus tents was not pretty. The showers looked like they were borrowed from the shower scene in the movie "M.A.S.H." Running water frequently ran out by mid-day and the port-a-potties had to be emptied twice daily. The air-conditioning unit faltered during the heat of the day and over-cooled at night. The amount of supplies and medicines we received overflowed the supply tent, forcing us to cover tons of supplies with tarps to protect our precious donations from the elements. Inventory was next to impossible. When the rainy season arrived early, in March, we had flooding, short circuits, and even an electrical fire.

Yet we persevered. The Israelis had set up an emergency hospital but they only stayed for two weeks. When they left, Medishare provided the only functioning critical care center in the entire country. Our operating rooms were performing fifty operations per day. At one point we had twenty spinal cord injury patients, with all of their complications. Our respirators sustained patients with tetanus. We even birthed two sets of triplets! Our prosthetics department fit more than two thousand limbs. Dr. Bob Gailey, who led that effort, swore we had served more amputees than we helped during the entire Vietnam War.

In the new hospital, one tent was reserved for adults. Children shared the second tent with operating and recovery rooms and intensive care units. There was a small, un-air conditioned tent that served as our emergency room and a second small tent for prosthetics. Two other tents served as our communications and logistics center. Outside our main tents, three small "tent cities" soon emerged – one for volunteer spill-over, one for patients' families and one for patients with suspected tuberculosis, who required isolation precautions.

Between patients, on my second tour of duty in February, my mind drifted frequently back to Janet – she had so resented my work in Haiti. It took the ordeal of her own suffering for her to learn why this work was so important. Thank God we'd reached peace on that by the end. Then there was the irony of the futility of her situation, and the impotency of medicine to help her. Back home medicine had become a business. Here, it was a profession again. We had a small army of doctors and nurses treating thousands of patients, helping every one of them, even if that help was simply pain relief and good nursing care. Here our business was giving hope to all the survivors stretched out in rows of cots, and the thousands more outside we would ultimately serve.

50
Limbo

The infant rescued from the rubble was officially known in the Jackson Memorial Hospital record system as "Unknown Infant Female." Unofficially, she was the instant darling of the nurses and staff of the Pedi-ICU. It didn't hurt that once the scabs on her abrasions fell off she was, in fact, impossibly cute. A little knit cap covered the small dent in her skull, the visible conse-quence of her healing skull fracture. She did all the things that two-month-old's do to endear themselves to us – sucking and burping and smiling and following us with their eyes. There was certain poignancy as she flapped her splinted forearms – a reminder of her ordeal; the one thing the Dr. Schneider missed on her initial exam and the one thing still keeping her in the ICU.

Whether it was a crush injury caused by falling concrete or the ever-stiffening post-mortem embrace of Marie-Ange, something compro-mised the circulation in her forearms, endangering the future use of her hands – a condition doctors call a "compartment syndrome." The ICU doctors found it in time, however, and two simple incisions relieved the pressure on her arteries and nerves. Soon, she was moving her fingers again and ready to be discharged to the regular pediatric unit.

There, even more nurses and staff fell in love with her – nurses would give up their breaks just to peer at her over her crib-rails. Many would cry, just at the sight of her – part tears of pain, having heard of the ordeal she went through and in part tears of joy for what she represented – a true miracle. At a time when uplifting stories were precious few, hers was one that gave hope. No need to question why this child got the miracle while hundreds of thousands of others equally deserving didn't – the important thing was that miracles do happen. Okay, granted rarely, but that's why they are miracles!

The Baby would have been the darling of an even larger circle of admirers had the hospital not surrounded her with a cloak of privacy. All the media that covered her resuscitation in Haiti were clamoring for updates and follow-up – begging for at least a still photo, all to no avail. The stated reason for this media blackout was that the hospital wanted to protect her privacy. Many suspected, however, that their real motivation was to avoid any controversy over the cost of providing critical care to an evacuated Haitian infant in a cash-strapped, tax-supported public hospital.

To complicate matters further, confusion reigned among all parties as to who was legally responsible for the child. Was it the hospital, the State Department, or Florida's Department of Children and Families? Until the issue of guardianship was resolved it would be impossible even to discharge her (ironically increasing the cost to taxpayers) let alone begin a search for her parents, whom we all assumed had died in the quake.

Meanwhile, Nadine and Junior subsisted in the abandoned car in the Hôpital Canapé Vert parking lot for a month after the quake. Junior scavenged daily for food and water, then returned to the wreckage of their former home, searching for mementoes of the baby. The rainy season started early – both a blessing and a curse – they could wash their clothes in collected rain and it flushed away the infernal dust, but it also flooded the parking lot. Soon mosquitoes plagued them. Junior eventually found a photo of Nadine and Jenny taken shortly after the baby's birth. He shared it with Kathie Klarreich. At least now they could prove they were the parents!

Kathie visited often, bringing food and reporting what news of Jenny she could glean from Miami (which was not much!). She also told their story to whoever would listen. Soon, other reporters started visiting also. They pooled their resources and purchased a tent for Junior and Nadine, allowing the couple to be able to relocate into a nearby encampment. With Kathie's encouragement, Junior and Nadine went to the U.S. Embassy to plead their case. Their plea was ignored. If they wanted to be rè-united with their daughter, the burden was on them to prove that she was, indeed, their daughter.

51
Another Miwak

It was the late afternoon in February 2010. I had just finished by my second post-quake tour of duty at the Medishare hospital. During my visits I had confined myself to work and the hospital, resisting the urge to tour the disaster zone. What good would it accomplish? Three weeks had passed since the quake. It had seemed like the media had saturated the story. Without anything to offer the destitute, I would only feel like a voyeur.

Ingrid, a former producer from CNN knew a thing or two about reporting the news and knew a lot about Haiti, insisted. She was daughter of a couple who ran an art gallery in Pétionville, which was how I got to know them. We bonded further as I nursed her father through his terminal illness.

"You need to see it, Art, with your own eyes," she warned me. "The true story is not being told"

So I went. What they called "tent cities" began about a kilometer from the airport and sprouted up wherever there was a patch of vacant land. Their name was a euphemism, giving the impression that the amenities we take for granted as part of city life – water, sanitation, security and shelter – would be there, even if houses were not. In reality, these were not tent cities, but rather makeshift encampments.

"It's scandalous," said Ingrid. "I mean, you can see a few tents distributed by the U.N. by the airport and near the presidential palace. That's where the media go. That's where it's convenient. But look at this! Mile upon mile of people living under sheets suspended from twigs. It's been three weeks. By now, someone should have done something."

Our itinerary, by coincidence, retraced the route Kathy Klarreich had taken the day she found Baby Jenny - through Cité Militaire, down Ave. Haile Selasec to Ave John Brown. We descended to Boulevard Harry Truman, skirting Cité Soleil. From there, we passed by the Champs Mars and Presidential Palace, The General Hospital and the Medical School, ascended Rue Canapé Vert, crossed over Delmas 48, and descended Rue Delmas, then returned to the airport, via Delmas 32.

My impressions from the air on my first trip post quake were confirmed. There was almost total devastation of neighborhoods rich, poor and in between. The exception was Cité Soleil, which survived relatively intact – a fortunate consequence of its flatness and lack of anything built of concrete. Every pillar of the Port au Prince social fabric was crushed, literally and figuratively. The Presidential Palace, all the ministries, including the Haitian equivalent of the Internal Revenue Service had been destroyed. There would be no taxes collected this year – there was no one to do it, no place to send them, no means of enforcement.

The medical school collapsed. Fortunately, the medical students were out on strike the day of the quake, so there were no casualties. The nursing school was totally destroyed. Their students – more conscientious or less politically active – all went to school that day. An entire class perished. The neighborhood of Canapé-Vert, where most professionals set-up their offices, was obliterated, buried by the collapse of the bidonville perched precariously above it

Randomly, an occasional edifice survived. Antique gingerbread houses stood out proudly from the rubble – most likely because wood shakes better than concrete. Father Luc's orphanage at Delmas 48 survived. The buildings to its right and left, however were now simply cavities in the earth.

The neighborhood of Delmas, the backbone of Haiti's working class, looked like it had been flattened by a steamroller. Yet here, and in every neighborhood we passed through, life had resumed. Amidst total destruction, market women were selling their wares while children played futbol in makeshift soccer fields. We passed hundreds of thousands of people carrying on. Three weeks into the disaster, Haitians were still clawing into the debris, trying to find loved ones.

"They see the earthquake as God's will," Ingrid murmured as she gazed out the car window, transfixed by the absurdity of it all. "A miwak! If it's God's will, then they must accept it's their fate. They search for good in it. It's a miracle, really…"

52
Loss of Comfort

One of the things that sustained Barth, Michel, Marie, myself and the other faculty associated with Medishare through the years were the medical students who "got it" - who learned from their time In Haiti that caring for the poor is the most noble calling of our profession. Medishare gave almost all of the thousands of students we brought to Thomonde a moving life experience, but most went on to traditional careers and traditional specialty choices. Their experiences in Haiti provided direct services and enriched their educational experience, but resulted in no long-term commitment to Haiti or global health.

There were, however, spectacular exceptions. The students who discovered congenital rubella in handicapped orphans all pursued careers in global health. Rick Spurlock, an early Medishare veteran, continued his commitment to Haiti through his residency and as an attending in emergency medicine at Emory University. He organized a Medishare chapter in Atlanta, recruiting students and faculty from both Emory and Morehouse schools of medicine and raising funds to build clinics in the remote Central Plateau communities of Bas Touribe and Casse.

I was pleased during my third tour of duty to be reunited with Amanda Harrington, a rehabilitation medicine specialist. Amanda was an early Medishare volunteer – as a medical student she visited Haiti three times. She continued her volunteerism through residency and now as a practicing physician. For several years she would give up a week of her vacation to precept our medical students during their trips to the Central Plateau. At the field hospital she finally had the opportunity to practice her own specialty – helping our amputees learn to walk again, rehabilitating spinal cord injury patients and caring for the wounds and bedsores of our sickest patients. She worked non-stop, stealing just a few hours to sleep each night, and giving our patients and us not just her technical expertise, but enthusiasm and compassionate care.

Another big success was Liz Greig. Liz entered medical school late, after a career working for an international philanthropy, choosing Miami over other prestigious schools because of the reputation Miami had earned, through Medishare, in global health. She traveled to Haiti as a first year student and made a life-time commitment. Upon return, her tales of her experiences convinced her parents, who unbeknownst to us, were considerably well off, to fund our Maternity Center in Marmont. Prior to the earthquake, she worked diligently with Barth to develop his plan for a national trauma network. When the earthquake struck, she postponed her planned wedding and put her fourth year electives on hold indefinitely to coordinate services between our field hospital and other providers.

"The Comfort is leaving!" Liz announced one morning as the lead agenda item during her morning call into our command center.

The Comfort was a U.S. Navy hospital ship, anchored two miles off of Port au Prince. With twelve operating rooms working round the clock, with surgeons, CAT scanners and one thousand beds, for six weeks, the Comfort had been a God-send – accepting our critical care patients, stabilizing them and sending them back to us or transferring them to hospitals in the States. Every day we had more and more patients like Baby Jenny – patients whose lives we knew we could save if only they had access to modern technology. The Comfort provided that technology and more

It had been six weeks now, however, and the Navy was getting anxious. The Comfort cost millions of dollars per day to operate and - given the magnitude of the disaster – there was no end of its need in sight. Compounding the dilemma, most of the staff of the Comfort were National Guardsman, pulled from their day jobs for earthquake-relief. They were anxious to return home. Given the Guard's commitments in Iraq and Afghanistan, there were no resources back home to replace them

"They claim they have a letter from the Haitian government that Haitian institutions are now back at full capacity," Liz said. "Therefore, the Comfort's services are no longer necessary."

"That's total B.S.!!" screamed Barth into the speakerphone. "We've got the only functioning trauma unit on the ground in the country and the only ICU beds. It will take weeks, if not months for Hôpital de la Paix and the General Hospital to build them. In the meantime, we're totally dependent on the Comfort for CAT scans and blood transfusions. Last night, you had a patient with blunt trauma to the head and a gunshot to the chest. The chest case burned through six units of blood. Without them we're cooked!"

"They claimed we can get blood from the General Hospital and that there's a functioning scanner up in Pétionville," answered Liz, meekly.

"Right!" responded Barth sarcastically. "So we load our patients with head trauma into tap-taps and send them through traffic up to Pétionville and back, praying they make it. Listen, we know the President (Preval), and he didn't sign that order, and we know the Minister of Health didn't sign it. What did they do – kidnap a secretary and force her to sign it as ransom? Listen, you tell them if they pull out, I'm going to go public and expose them for the two-faced hypocrites that they are! They loved it when the reporters of CNN and ABC news visited them!"

"Uh… That's above my pay grade, Dr. Green…"

"Don't worry, Liz, I'll be on the plane down tomorrow to bash a few heads."

Barth's threat to go public bought us two weeks time, plus a small grant from U.S. Agency for International Development to upgrade our hospital, with better operating rooms, a CAT scanner, and a blood bank. The Navy abandoned its ploy to credit the Comfort's departure to "mission accomplished." Instead, they said the ship needed to refuel. It never returned.

The departure of the Comfort was just one very visible sign of several international agencies either pulling out or scaling back. The Israelis had packed up their field hospital and flew home. The Red Cross and UNICEF, claiming to be unprepared for a disaster on this order of magnitude, were almost invisible on the ground. To make matters worse, the rainy season started early – drenching our campsite, flooding our lodging tent, muddying our roads and raising the specter of malaria and dengue.

The quake and its aftermath were yet another example of how the laws of thermodynamics apply not just to physics but also to biology, economics, and politics. There is an inexorable tendency to randomness and disorder. One must put enormous energy into systems to maintain order and some of that energy is inevitably dissipated as heat – a phenomenon known as entropy. The quake was the ultimate entropic event – the release of destructive force in a thirty five second time span that had been gradually building in the fault-line for centuries – entropy to the 11th power. The second law of thermodynamics - the natural tendency towards randomness and disorder – the law of entropy, also applied to the relief effort. It would take an enormous amount of energy, time, and money just to get back to a pre-quake level of order and organization. The international organizations had the money, but lacked the energy. If there was hope, it would have to come from the people themselves.

For most *Vodouisants*, the metaphysical significance of the quake was clear - the quake would bring Haiti to its crossroads. Maybe, just maybe, Haiti's turbulent past would die with the earthquake's victims and a new Haiti would be born. Perhaps the self-discipline and motivation to lead a good life helping others, purely because it's the right thing to do, so central to *Vodou*, would finally prevail over the cynical real-politick that dominated the capital and an economy in which millions of poor suffered daily misery so that those who lived well, could live very well indeed...

From this perspective, the quake was part of *Bondye's* plan – the good of it only for Him to know. It was another mountain to climb, one more obstacle to overcome. When the rains came, the *Vodouisants* undressed, stepped out of their tents and lean-to's, and for the first time in weeks, washed themselves clean. *Mesi, Ampil, Bondye! Lapli Tombe!* Praise be to God! The rains are falling! We are clean again. Our sins are washed away. We can begin again. A second baptism...

53
The Bandwagon

A month after the earthquake, it seemed that everyone wanted to climb onto the Medishare field hospital bandwagon. Our dean, Dr. Pascal Goldschmidt made an overnight visit, serving both as a cardiology consultant and a translator. Upon return, he declared The Miller School of Medicine's response to the disaster was "our finest hour." Following his visit, a parade of UM administrators and associate deans made pilgrimage to the hospital, as well as departmental chairs and members of the faculty, some of whom did several tours of duty.

Volunteers came from as far as California. We provided them with transportation to Haiti and back to Miami and free lodging in our tents in exchange for eight days of voluntary service. Dr. Samantha Madhosingh, a child psychologist from Washington D.C, recruited more than six hundred mental health professionals over the internet to address the mental health needs of quake victims, their families, and, as we soon discovered, our volunteers.

Samantha organized the volunteers into teams including Kreyol and non-Kreyol mental health professionals and made sure they all used the same methodology to address the grieving and stress caused by the quake. In retrospect, it should have been obvious that a catastrophe of this magnitude would cause significant mental health problems. To her credit and ours, Samantha and Medishare were among the few who planned proactively for the mental health of the victims.

As it turned out, not just the Haitians needed counseling. Most volunteers had an overwhelming positive experience. For some, however, the stress of caring for critically ill patients, the emotional strain of losing the lives of patients they worked so hard to save, and the sheer order of magnitude of the tragedy caused them to snap -- raging and displacing their anger at the death and suffering we were all dealing with onto seemingly trivial inconveniences, like waiting in line for supplies or an airplane flight home.

By the end of the first month, the number of cases of earthquake – related trauma began to subside. The hospital took over general trauma and general hospital needs. Patients who had never seen a doctor before showed up in our emergency room with complaints from the sublime to the ridiculous, lured by the possibility, for the first time, of free, quality health care.

All this success, however, came at a price. The cost of flying in and lodging volunteers was very expensive, as were the operating costs of the hospital. Moreover, with Haitian hospitals destroyed, Haitian doctors and nurses needed work. Soon, grumblings surfaced – why weren't we developing a Haitian work force? Why were we delivering free care to everyone? How could Haiti sustain the kind of care we were delivering?

54
Resurrection

For the first time in Haiti's history, Carnival was cancelled in 2010. The weeks leading up to Lent are usually time for organizing, planning, building floats, making masks and costumes, culminating in the riotous all night bacchanalia which is Mardi Gras – a time to put one's tribulations aside for a while and celebrate life. Even in the worst of the bad times, demonstrations, political theatre, class differences, and the daily misery of life among the poor were briefly replaced during Carnival by music, dance, and spectacle. Not this year, however. This year the focus was on Ash Wednesday. Ashes to ashes, dust to dust. Remember man that thou art mortal. Not that this particular year, we needed any reminders.

Memorial services were held throughout the country. Prayers for the dead were offered, along with hope that families and loved ones would one day be reunited. Remember that the *Vodouisant* thinks of death differently. Death is a crossing from this life to paradise in Guinea. Its freedom from the miseries and injustice and an opportunity to be reunited with family and friends.

Resurrection is a very real phenomenon for the *Vodouisant*. The Catholics and Protestants talk about resurrection. Vodouisants see it and feel it. Victims of the zombie curse die and are buried, then are resurrected, albeit to a life of slavery. At the end of the *cris*, the climax of the Vodou ceremony, Vodouisants collapse, die for an instant – their spirits unite with Lwa and their bodies apparently lifeless, are then resurrected by the joy of the spiritual encounter.

Haiti as we knew it died January 12, 2010. Its *cris* lasted not an instant, but months. During that time, its own government and international agencies tried to reanimate it, but failed. It was too overwhelming a disaster, they claimed. Immediately after the quake, "cluster groups" were organized to plan the recovery. Consisting of representatives of the government, international agencies, and NGO's, they attempted to address the major post-quake issues such as health, housing, water, and sanitation. With no one in charge, however, their plans soon dissolved into speculative philosophy accomplishing nothing. Three months after the earthquake, more than two billion dollars had been donated or pledged to Haiti, most of it from concerned individuals. Best estimates are that between one to twenty percent actually trickled down to the Haitian people – at least by the time in early March when the government declared the recovery period over and the rebuilding phase about to begin.

Agencies bickered about how to solve key problems. Early on, it was determined there were not enough tents to distribute, so tarps were handed out instead. All told, only about half the people who needed shelter got it – the rest improvised with sheets and blankets. A satisfactory solution to the problem of sanitation was hotly debated. Latrines obviously, would help and organizing a corps of latrines-diggers would create jobs. It was claimed, however, that there just wasn't enough cleared space, and no one ever took charge. The latrines were never dug.

There was also much give and take in the media and among the government as to how to rebuild. Should the capital be moved? It was, after all, sitting on a fault line. How big should the capital be? How could the homeless best be transitioned to permanent housing? Should the plan be "centralized" or "de-centralized?" These discussions dissipated much heat, but generated little light and no action.

Lip service was given to the sovereignty of the Haitian government, but few in the international community trusted them or empowered them. The Haitians, in response, soon asked questions as to how the international agencies were spending money and making decisions. A backlash against NGO's soon developed. Graffiti on walls declared *Au ba* NGO's! ("Down with NGO's") Such are the consequences of a top-down humanitarian response.

If there was hope, it came from the people themselves. Like a mambo reviving herself after a cris, the people began the resurrection of the new Haiti. In the tent cities, natural leaders emerged and transformed the camps into communities – organizing work-groups and finding solutions for accessing healthcare, clean water, sanitation, and jobs. About half of the homeless voted with their feet and made their way back to communities where they had once lived. Thomonde now has 25,000 more people than it did before the earthquake. Hopefully, they find not just to a refuge, but the world-view and way of life that sustained their ancestors for centuries.

Romel Joseph's first attempts to play the violin were both clumsy and painful – his left hand, still swollen from its injury and surgery could barely wrap around the violin's neck. Resurrecting the strength and agility of his fingers to anything approaching his pre-quake skill would prove to be an arduous task. By April, however, he felt well enough to return to Haiti, to oversee the clearing of rubble from the site of his destroyed school.

55
Proof

Back in Miami, I received a call in my office from a Haitian – American attorney, Mr. Mark Lapointe.

"Dr. Fournier – I've seen on the news all the wonderful things you're doing and I want to know if I can help!"

The legalisms surrounding Baby Jenny had grown increasingly frustrating. No one seemed to be in charge. Several entities, including Jackson Memorial Hospital, Florida's Department of Children and Families and the State Department seemed to be simultaneously trying to control the child's fate. At the same time, they abdicated themselves from any decision that might have adverse consequences, either in terms of liability or media relations. To make matters worse, as rumors that the child might have surviving parents surfaced, the media, sensing another miracle story, clamored for access. They called incessantly to see if I could, at best, convince the hospital that the press had a right to see the child and tell her story or, at least, snap a picture. The child had long recovered from her most serious injuries, yet languished in the hospital, with shift-nurses serving, through no fault of their own, as poor substitutes for an actual parent. I suggested Mark talk with the Haitian Immigrant Advocacy Center about getting himself appointed as the child's guardian. I had no idea if this would even be remotely possible, but figured there was nothing to lose.

Mark thanked me for the idea and said goodbye. I heard nothing for several weeks, then the attorney for the hospital called to inform me that Mark LaPointe had been named legal guardian of the baby. She would be placed in the custody of Florida's Department of Children and Families and discharged to a foster home, while claims of parenthood were investigated.

Mark was intrigued CNN's report on a Port au Prince couple, Nadine and Junior Alexis, who claimed to be the parents. While I was skeptical of their story, Mark understood that it was in the best interests of the baby to check it out. He tracked down Junior and Nadine and interviewed them in Kreyol. Their story seemed plausible enough. Thinking like a lawyers, he realized he could not represent the child and the couple who claimed to be her parents. He, therefore, called on another attorney, Bob Martinez to represent Junior and Nadine. Miami is a community frequently fractured along ethnic divides and one would be hard-pressed to find many examples of Cuban-American and Haitian-American collaboration. Bob Martinez and Mark LaPointe turned out to be the exception.

Junior and Nadine had been fighting depression for weeks. Their home had been destroyed. They had lost many relatives. They had lost Marie-Ange their babysitter. Junior had lost his livelihood, nightclub singing, at least for the foreseeable future. And they knew their daughter was alive in Miami. They received occasional word of her well being from Kathie and other reporters. They, however, were stuck in a tent city and had no prospects of being reunited with their daughter. It was understandable, therefore, that they when a Cuban-American attorney, Bob, showed up with an offer to help, they responded with a certain degree of skepticism.

It's difficult to describe with word the conditions of the encampments five months after the earthquake. Sun and rain had long decomposed the water-repellant of the few officially distributed tents. Torrential daily rains turned the small paths separating the tents to rivers of mud. Flooding soaked the floors, which seepage from tent walls and rook soaked everything else. Clothes hung out to dry – clotheslines strung between tents hardly ever dried. U.N. soldiers gathered by their trucks, at the corners of encampment, guns at the ready. Without a birth certificate or testimonials from eyewitnesses, proving paternity (or in actuality, maternity) would be difficult.

Bob latched on to a family re-unification program run by the International Red Cross that ran DNA tests to establish family ties. Bob called them. Yes, they would be willing to do DNA testing. Bob posed the same question to Junior and Nadine. Without hesitation, they agreed. All the test required was a swab from Nadine's cheek and one from Jenny's. Weeks passed. Junior and Nadine prayed daily, hoping to be reunited with their daughter. Finally, the word arrived – the match was positive. What the baby's parents had affirmed all along was confirmed by science – with 99.99 percent accuracy, Nadine was Jenny's mother!

There was still, however, the problem of reuniting the child with her parents – the child being in Miami and the parents in Haiti. From the moment the quake struck, the State Department was dead set against allowing Haitians into the country. Once the test results came back, Bob and Mark could work as a team, since they shared a common goal – bringing the family back together again.

The judges they faced proved surprisingly sympathetic. Bob, armed with the DNA test proving Nadine was the baby's mother, as well as a strong case that Jenny might die if faced to return to the unsanitary conditions of the camp, filed for humanitarian parole.

The metaphysical questions I grappled with during Janet's illness returned once again. What if Barth hadn't been so determined to set up a hospital in Haiti immediately after the quake? What if Kathie Klarreich hadn't fallen in love with Haiti some two decades earlier, hadn't ventured into Canapé Vert at the exact moment Jenny was excavated or didn't have the where-with-all to bring her to our hospital? What if the two Karens hadn't been there? What if Barth hadn't had wealthy connections with airplanes? What if there weren't the two lawyers in Miami--one Haitian-American, one Cuban-American--willing to work together, pushing the system simply to do the right thing? It was hard to explain how Baby Jenny was returned to her parents by random collision of molecules. I had to believe the story was a vindication of the Vodou creed – of the primacy of family, obligation to always do the right thing, to love and help one another, and the meaning we can find in all life's events. The power of hope and even the possibility of the intercession of the Lwa!

On April 5th, 2010, a federal judge in Miami granted Nadine and Junior humanitarian parole. Bob and Mark flew down to Haiti the following day on the Project Medishare plane, returning on the turnaround flight along with a plane full of Project Medishare volunteers. The parents were united with their daughter that afternoon – their prayers answered, their faith and hope affirmed. The courts have extended humanitarian parole for two years. It is unclear at this writing if, after that, the family will return to Haiti. Bob is advocating that they stay here. I view that choice with ambivalence. I certainly don't want them to return to the squalor that is now Port au Prince just because Miami is more materially well off does not mean it is spiritually or metaphysically superior.

In any event, in the interim, I can visit often. Jenny is beautiful, bright, and alert – advanced for her age. I think she sees me as a funny looking uncle. I always leave, however, with a gentle admonishment to Nadine and Junior.

"Li fok Pa bliye li Ayitién.,"

"She must not forget she's Haitian."

56
Muddied Water

The almost universal response of friends and colleagues when they heard of the outbreak of cholera in Haiti in the fall of 2010 was, "Oh, no! Not another curse on that God-Forsaken country!" With cholera as the fourth horseman, following AIDS, rebellion and the earthquake, the theory that that Haiti is cursed" theory gained new credibility. The truth however, is that most of Haiti's curses, cholera included, are the consequences of the actions of men. Similar to the flooding in Gonaives three years before, errors of omission and commission not just exacerbated the epidemic but contributed to its cause and explosive spread.

Given the lack of clean water and adequate sanitation in Haiti, it was no surprise that a waterborne illness became epidemic. In fact, could be considered a miwak it didn't emerge sooner. Death from diarrhea was the most common cause of death among children, even prior to the earthquake. When Medishare first arrived in the Central Plateau, one in five children died before their fifth birthday – usually from infantile diarrhea. By 2009, our community health program had cut that figure in half. One of the reasons for our success was our health agents teaching about and distributing packets of oral rehydration therapy – a simple combination of sugar and salt that allows fluids to be absorbed by even inflamed or damaged intestines. Modern medicine doesn't like to admit it but Gatorade this homespun can save more lives than antibiotics.

If the truth be known, however cholera had nothing to do with the earthquake. There were two mysteries to this latest scourge: why did cholera emerge where it did? and what caused it?. The first cases were reported in small villages near the mouth of the Artibonite, Haiti's largest river, just north of St. Marc, about sixty miles east of Port au Prince – a pastoral setting of small villages surrounded by irrigation canals and rice paddies. On October 20th, small clinics there reported being overwhelmed by about fifty patients with fever, vomiting and explosive diarrhea. There were also reports of people found dead by the side of the road - a macabre tribute to just how quickly this disease could suck the life out of its victims. In fact, although public health officials in Haiti and global health authorities around the world restrained themselves, awaiting official confirmation to avoid panic, we all knew that cholera was the only gastro-intestinal disease that could kill that quickly. By the second day, the regional public hospital in Saint Marc was overwhelmed, with over five hundred cases and more than 100 deaths. The next day, as tests confirmed the disease was, indeed, cholera, cases were also reported in Mirebalais, at the headquarters of the Artibonite.

Sanitation had long been neglected in the Artibonite and the people routinely bathe and get their drinking water from the river and its tributaries. The outbreak occurred at the end of the rainy season, when the water table, at its crest, floods the makeshift latrines. All of this, however, begs the question – why there?

The Haitians of course, knew right away – the reason was the Nepalese MINUSTAH camp in Mirebalais. MINUSTAH denied it, of course, in spite of investigative journalists from the Associated Press photographing raw sewage dumping from the latrines into a tributary of the Artibonite. Cholera is endemic to Nepal. When tests showed the strain causing the epidemic was endemic to "South Asia", the U.N. countered that none of the soldiers they tested carried the strain. Ultimately, a French epidemiologist confirmed what the Haitians had affirmed all along.

To the Haitians the origin of the epidemic was important for two reasons. First, having already been stigmatized unjustly for bringing AIDS into the world, they were not going to be blamed for cholera. More importantly, the U.N. has to be held accountable. Resentment of the U.N. had been brewing for years among Haitians, fueled by reports of troops exploiting Haitian women and children. The Haitians knew they were dumping raw sewage into the river, but no one listened. Literally and figuratively, the United Nations were crapping on the people of Haiti. The least they could do was to create adequate sanitation in their own camps.

If humans cause Haiti's curses they can also cure them. Medishare's presence in the Central Plateau, just to the north of the Artibonite, as well as its decade-long experience with community health, made it ideally suited to respond. Marie deployed community health workers from Thomonde to the Artibonite. She directed volunteers and supplies from our hospital in Port au Prince to the hospital in St. Marc, arming them with bullhorns and packets of oral rehydration therapy, as well as donations of bleach and soap. They initiated a community education campaign about cholera, in small village at a time. Within a week of the outbreak Medishare and Paul Farmer's group, Partners in Health, opened a

Cholera Treatment Center in Mirebalais. Two months after the out-break, we had treated more than six thousand patients, with only forty deaths.

And so the Haitian people endure. The earthquake didn't de-stroy them. Cholera won't either. They refuse to despair. While they live, they hope.

57
Crossroads

It took an immense tragedy to return the world's attention to Haiti. Never mind that much of the attention the disaster created was simply morbid curiosity, salted with disaster voyeurism. The way the Haitian people responded – with patience, resilience and en-durance will hopefully awaken decision makers from their zombie curse and create a resolve to finally get it right this time. "No more band aids for Haiti!" Are the rallying cry of those, Haitian and non-Haitian, who care about the country and its people?

Such optimism however is probably naïve. First, Haiti's fifteen minutes of fame are already over. The media has moved on to earthquakes in Chile and Turkey, health care reform, the oil spill in the Gulf and the presidential elections. Appropriations from the U.S. to rebuilding Haiti will be controlled by the party in power in the House of Representatives. That party will change as early as January.

Second, even with sufficient funding, there is no precedent as to how to proceed. William Easterly, in "The White Man's Burden," writes eloquently on the two great scourges of modern life – the death and misery caused by poverty and the amount of money thrown at the problem by international philanthropy, to no effect. If "The White Man's Burden" is not sufficiently sobering, pick up David Rieff's "A Bed for the Night," in which the humanitarian cause is exposed as a front for international "realpolitik." While one can debate, Rieff's premise from a theoretical perspective, there is a strong dose of truth in his account of how humanitarian aid has played out in Haiti in the past.

Finally, there is no consensus concerning recovery, among Haitians or among international agencies. More than nine hundred agencies are registered to work in Haiti, ranging from small missionary groups through NGO's like Project Medishare to governmental agencies, contractors, and international relief organizations. Some have good working relationships with the Haitian government, most do not. Many have hidden religious (i.e. missionary), political (i.e. USAID), or economic (i.e. the so-called "Beltway Bandit" consultants) agendas. Few have Haitians in leadership positions. The traditional, top-down international approach seems doomed to failure. Likewise, with its infrastructure in shambles, it's unlikely that, even with $2 billion worth of pledges, the Haitian government could pull off rebuilding on its own.

There is, in Haiti, a tradition of the *"konbit"* – a communal workforce that comes together for common cause – usually planting and harvesting or building a home. In the tent cities after the quake, konbits formed spontaneously. Out of these konbits, natural leaders emerged, local problems were identified and solved. These konbits should be funded with seed money, even as the encampments are dismantled and their residents relocated. Individuals should also be funded via microfinance to create a sustainable rural middle class.

Rural Haiti needs to be re-invented even more than Port au Prince. Those half-million people who returned to their ancestral towns and villages after January 12 should be encouraged to stay there. Thomonde will certainly change with the arrival of thousands of people, many who have never lived there or who have only distant memories. But creating jobs in health and education as well as agri-culture can help build a new infrastructure of safe water, sanitation, schools, and clinics. Haiti can recover one community at a time. To their credit, those designing the National Recovery Plan seem to understand this. They've made decentralization and revitalization of the rural economy cornerstones of Haiti's recovery plan.

International agencies and NGOs cannot just be funders. People of good will who want to help resurrect Haiti need to be thoroughly versed in its unique history, culture, language, and religion. Moreover, they will need to overcome the class and race stereotypes that taint pretty much all of us and bond with the Haitian people they are trying to help. This will involve getting out of Port au Prince on a regular basis, at the very least and at best, living with the people, experiencing their miseries and joys for extended periods of time, discovering who the natural leaders of each community are and who's solving problems on a local level.

The earthquake brought Haiti to a metaphysical crossroads. The old Haiti, a nation dominated by an unlanded aristocracy in Port au Prince and an African-esque peasantry in the countryside, died on January 12, 2010. On one hand much of the wealth of the elite was destroyed by the quake. On the other, the historic trends of migration from the countryside to the city have been reversed. The values of the Vodouisant, so necessary for survival in a harsh environment, are to be found in their purest form in rural Haiti. Those values will be tested by the influx of city-folks and well-intentioned foreigners who will expose Haitians to the materialism and insanity of the modern world. Time will tell whether the Vodouisant worldview will survive greater exposure to the world at large. I hope so. Baron Samedi brought an entire country to the crossroads – from past to future, from life to death and hopefully back again.

58
The Brass Band

After five months of chaos in the capital, by June things were stable enough for Medishare to resume its student-faculty trips to Thomonde. Not that things were necessarily better in Port au Prince – most people were still living in tents, sanitation was awful and a premature rainy season added new dimensions to misery there. The number of trauma cases coming into our field hospital, however, plummeted to pre-earthquake levels, allowing us to shift some of our focus back to our original programs.

From January until June, Marie had performed a seemingly impossible balancing act, keeping Medishare's programs in the Central Plateau running while dealing with the daily drama at the field hospital in Port au Prince. Our students, moved by the plight of Haiti, were clamoring to do something, but in all honesty, their skill set was more suited to the primary care and prevention programs we ran in the Central Plateau than the trauma programs we developed post-quake in Port au Prince. Plus, in my heart-of-hearts, I yearned to return to rural Haiti, my Vodou Shangri-La.

The first day of this particular trip, the students and faculty made home visits with our health agents. Days Two through Four we participated in mobile clinics in the remote communities of *Cheryval, Cay Epin* and *Ti Casse.* The final day, we were scheduled to do school health physicals in *Casse-La Hoye* – a forty five minute drive from the Medishare headquarters in Thomonde.

To my usual repertoire of vignettes over breakfast, I added tales of the earthquake – Medishare and the Miller's School's heroic response, as well as the miracle of Baby Jenny and her reunion with her parents. Most of all, I shared with them the lessons of spirit – fortitude, resilience, patience and hope that I've learned from the Haitian people.

As we were heading out of Thomonde, we passed a church with a brass band assembling in front. Clearly, a funeral was about to take place. Another death. Baron Samedi – 300,000 souls in Port au Prince were not enough? I explained to my students this Haitian rite of passage – a coming to the crossroads, heralded by trumpets and slide trombones. When we returned several hours later, the funeral was still in progress. In fact, the mourners marched by Medishare's headquarters. I excused myself from a discussion with my students about a patient we had seen earlier in the day, to stand at the curbside as the coffin and mourners passed. One more death to remember, and a reminder that death will one day claim all of us, myself included. Baron Samedi holds all the cards.

Socrates is a man

All men are mortal…

So why fight it? In certain instances, we shouldn't. Instead, we should ease it. At the very end, death was a blessing for Janet, as it was for hundreds of quake victims, for whom our interventions at the field hospital only prolonged the inevitable. Sex and death are the engines of evolutionary progress, so we might as well accept it as an inevitable fact of life. At the same time, premature death, painful death and messy death are unequivocal tragedies – something not just doctors should fight against but all of us, by ameliorating or eliminating those conditions – poverty, inequality, injustice, war to name a few – that give Baron Samedi the upper hand. The lessons from Janet's illness and Haiti's earthquake are one and the same. No man is an island. Do not ask for whom the brass band plays. It plays for thee.

59
Star-gazing

My days in Thomonde start and end with meditation. Long before dawn, the braying of mules, the crowing of roosters and the claptrap of cowbells awaken me. I've slept soundly and look forward to my few hours of solitude before the workday begins. It's a time to meditate, reflect, and to write. As the sun rises it illuminates a painting of Erzilie/Athena/Aphrodite/the Virgin holding a child. I had bought the painting on one of my first trips to Haiti, thinking it was "neat," but not fully appreciating its significance. The Mother and Child were painted as icons, almost in a Byzantine style. There were curious geometric patterns all around the borders and in each corner - *"veve"* - abstract symbols of the goddess/ *Lwa Erzili* – a heart with a cross set upon it: the heart for love and the cross for suffering. Back then, I marveled at how the artist – someone Haitian art scholars term a "primitive" – could adopt a style that originated in Byzantium. I also wondered what meaning could there be in all this syncretism. Now, having lived through the struggles of Janet, Nadine and Baby Jenny, I get it: the primacy of family; the sacred bond of mother and child; the bond that links the chain of generations of humanity and source of all noble human attributes; the wisdom in love; the love in wisdom and the inextricable relationship between love, suffering and salvation. All these concepts, idealized, abstracted and conveyed to me by the talent of the artist. Janet now was *Erzili* and *Erzili* Janet – the mother of my children, the heart, a symbol of her love and the cross, simultaneously a symbol of her suffering and her passage through the crossroads.

This is now my world of the spirit – those intangible thoughts, emotions, ideas, insights, memories and abstractions that exist only in my mind. There is so much meaning in everything, even gobs of paint on a wooden plank. More to the point, here was a people that gave meaning to my life – a place where I could still make a difference. I conclude my meditation with thoughts of my departed ancestors – my wonderful grandparents, my stern, but hard-working father, and, finally, Janet: the carefree times when we first met, her devotion to our children, the joy she took in teaching and her valiant struggle against her cruel fate.

The muted sounds of women, our housekeepers, outside my door tell me that coffee and breakfast have been brought for me and my workday is about to begin. I start my day, while I sip my coffee, by "rounding" in my mind on my patients who've died – Regina, who chose getting pregnant with Lupus, knowing it might kill her (it did); Mary, who loved me as if I were her grandson, in spite of the fact that it took me seventeen years to figure out her headaches were caused by a slowly leaking aneurysm; and, of course, Regis and all the others who died of AIDS in the early days. I finish with a remembrance of the victims of the quake and cholera, particularly those buried in the unmarked graves. Janet's suffering sensitized me to their suffering – each one a unique individual, snatched away by that trichoter, Samedi.

That particular day after two cups of Haitian coffee and a plate of spaghetti Kreyol, I mingled with the health agents as we all prepared to begin our day's assignments. Marie organized us all, making sure that the agents doing vaccinations had ice in their coolers, that the agents doing direct observed therapy had their documentation forms and that the traditional birth attendants had their birthing kits. Watching the health agents as they prepared to depart, it was impossible not to take tremendous pride on what we've been able to achieve in Thomonde. Marie took me aside that day, seeing the quiet satisfaction in my eyes and whispering "Dr. Fournier, you've been away too long."

Workdays in Thomonde pass. But in the evening, after the health workers have turned in their forms, and, after the medical students have "de-briefed," it's my habit, weather permitting, to set aside a little time for star-gazing. On a clear night, there's probably no place better on Earth to contemplate the universe than Thomonde. Without street lights, electricity, or the loom of another town or city to dim the effect, the entire Milky Way arches over my head. The planets and constellations assume a brilliance here that one could not even imagine in Miami. From time immemorial humans – not just philosophers, theologian and scientists, but "everymen" – have looked to the heavens for inspiration and for answers.

Stargazing is the original game of "connect the dots." That capacity to connect the dots – to find meaning in seeming randomness is a unique human trait, refined by eons of natural selection – helps us survive and flourish as a species. That drive to search for meaning ingrained in all of us is the well-spring of science, philosophy and Vodou. The problem is, each of these quests for meaning provides different, and frequently, contradicting answers.

For scientists, star-gazing has been particularly productive, assisting the ancients with the pragmatic business of navigation and moderns with knowledge of the nature of the solar systems, the law of gravity, the theory of relativity and the origins of the universe. The value of star-gazing by philosophers and theologians is more difficult to assess. On the one hand, pondering the heavens probably contributed to the concepts of order in the universe and the prime mover – conceptual arguments in favor of the existence of a Supreme Being. On the other hand, speculation about the heavens, unbridled by the facts provided by science, set back the quest for knowledge and wisdom for centuries, gave rise to the pseudoscience of Astrology and created a rift between science and religion that persists to this day.

But what about "everyman"? The people of Thomonde are the quintessential "everymen." For the *Vodouisants* of Thomonde, the stars are not only an inescapably intense reality, but are alive with meaning. Where we see Gemini, they see *Marassa* (the Vodou twin Lwa). Where we see Drago, they see *Damballah*, the snake-god. Where we see Venus, they see Erzilie. Where we see the Milky Way, they see a heavenly host of *Ti-Lwa*, waiting for prayers, waiting to intercede on our behalf. For the *Vodouisant*, if it moves, it's alive, at least alive with meaning. Stars twinkle and planets move, so they are living creatures, like us. This search for meaning in everything is at the heart of Vodou. I think, however, this essence of Vodou is there in all of us, Vodouisant or not. Furthermore, that search for meaning is not an end in itself, but really a means to an end – that end being wisdom.

It's always astounded me how even the poorest of Haitians aspire to wisdom. Philosophy is not learned in the classroom and forgotten after the test, but learned on the knee of your grandparents and then lived for the rest of your life. In a country and culture where few can afford the luxury of schooling, wisdom is passed from generation to the next. Wisdom is so revered in Haiti that peasants not infrequently name their children after philosophers – Voltaire, Rousseau, Marc-Aurele and Aristide (Aristotle) are all common Haitian names. So Thomonde is not just a great place for stargazing, it's probably my best hope to figure this all out – to find meaning in Janet's suffering and death as well as the death of hundreds of thousands of innocent earthquake and cholera victims.

I certainly wouldn't be able to sort things through in Miami, where the stars are dimmed to imperceptibility by the lights of the city, where the meaning of life is lost in the mundane details of modernity and the quest for wisdom is relegated to a small circle of academics, hoping to get some papers out of it. So here I sit in Thomonde, gazing at the stars and straddling two worlds, the world of Science and the world of Spirit. Can these worlds possibly be reconciled?

I've been blessed or perhaps cursed with unique experiences – a career in academic medicine that taught me both the power and limitations of science, work in Haiti that had opened my eyes to an alternative world view and the gut-wrenching emotional experiences of the pre-mature loss of my wife, the earthquake and now cholera.

The years since Janet's passing have taken the edge off the emotional side of that experience, allowing me, good *Vodouisant* that I'm becoming, to now stop and try and find meaning in it: not just the meaning of her life, suffering and death, but what it means for all of us. The casualties of the earthquake and the cholera outbreak take those speculations to a whole different dimension. We as individuals and as a species are fragile, vulnerable and exquisitely mortal. What wisdom can we distill from the worlds of Science and Spirit, and the fact that we are all mortal and that most of us will either suffer ourselves or witness it in loved ones? In spite of Aquinas' assertions that there was no conflict between faith and reason, science, philosophy and theology have been light years apart on the meaning of life, death and suffering for centuries. Perhaps the answers I'm seeking will never be found in these disparate ways of thinking. Perhaps the experiences of caring for Janet through her ordeal and the example she set, as well as the example set by the survivors of the earthquake are the real path to wisdom.

The belief in life everlasting persists in most of us, in spite of the fact that there is overwhelming evidence that the brain, mind and spirit are one, because hope is one of those intangibles most of us need to live. In fact, the Haitians believe strongly that "Lespwa fe viv." Hope is a prerequisite for not only our individual survival, but also the survival of our species.

Such speculations on a starry night in Thomonde are entertaining, if kept in perspective. Certainly, after witnessing Janet's suffering and the suffering of millions of Haitians, the belief in a benevolent God that rewards the good and those that suffer is a comforting speculation. I also now understood why my Italian mother and grandparents venerated the saints, as Vodouisants worship the *Lwa*, hoping for miracles. In truth, however, such beliefs are most likely simply products of our imagination. Imagination is a wonderful thing – it certainly is the source of our creativity and, as such, has helped us to survive and flourish as a species. However, not everything we imagine is necessarily real, as much as we might like it to be. No, better that we should make the work of rewarding the good, healing the sick and alleviating suffering our own. That's why I'm here in Thomonde.

We are, by our biologic nature, intelligent and social beings. None of us has the capacity to live totally alone. That's what's so appealing about working here in Thomonde – our interdependency here is so apparent, starting with the close bonds between parents and children and extending throughout the village and the commune. When houses need to be built or fields cleared, the Thomondois organize themselves into konbits, communal work groups. If a *malad* (sick person) becomes too weak to walk, neighbors will carry him or her to the hospital, tend his fields or feed her children. In fact, it's a paradox. The harshness of the Thomonde physical environment is exactly what brings out the positive social traits embodied in its *Vodouisants*. Someday Samedi will come stalking. It's better not to have to face him alone.

It's clear to me now, like the clarity of the sky above me. Like the infinite numbers of points on a finite line, our limited, mortal souls have limitless capacity for discovery, knowledge, imagination and creativity. Our spirits are daily at the crossroads. We can travel back in time to our childhood with our memories and, through our scientific knowledge, to the very origins of the universe. We can also travel to the future, albeit with a little less certainty, making reasonable estimates and predictions of everything from the weather and what our lives will be like the next day, to when life on Earth will end. Through art and writing, we can express our souls and give them a tangible, material presence. We can even achieve some semblance of immortality, through the remembrances of family and friends, and the legacies, material and spiritual, that we leave behind.

To the Haitians, *Bondye*, the great god who made the Earth and moves the sun, the moon and the planets, is a creator, not in the western sense of a supreme wizard who created the universe out of nothing, but a creator in the sense of an artist. Take the sky I'm studying. For the Haitians, it's God's canvas. To be an artist, therefore, is to be like God. No wonder Haiti is a nation of artists! But *Bondye* is also a benevolent, loving Spirit, welcoming the souls of departed *Vodouisants* back to Guinea and interceding on behalf of supplicants who approach Him through the Lwa. To do good is, therefore, to be like *Bondye*. Our communal life here in Thomonde is God's moral canvas. No wonder Haiti is a nation of *Vodouisants*. Here, God's work truly is our own. If hope is to exist, we must create it ourselves.

Epilogue

April 2012:

Baby Jenny celebrated her second birthday last November with no long-term consequences of her ordeal. In fact, she seems a perfect child in every way. Nadine and Junior, however, are having difficulty adjusting to life in Miami." It's not home!" they say." The people here are just not as friendly and we miss the family we left behind". Their two years' humanitarian parole expires in two months. They probably will not be able to return to Haiti, however, as there is, in fact, no place for them to return to. More than two years after the quake about a half million people are still living in tent cities, including those members of their families who survived. Three waves of cholera have scoured the countryside and a fourth is anticipated with this summer's rainy season. At this writing more than 7000 patients have died from cholera and 500,000 have been infected. If intensive interventions are not rapidly implemented there may be up to 70,000 deaths by the time of the sixth wave.

The elections scheduled for the fall of 2010 were first postponed and then contested. These political issues have delayed the implementation of a national plan agreed upon by the Haitian government and international donors in the months following the earthquake, under the umbrella of the Interim Haiti Relief Committee. This plan emphasized decentralization and job creation and the resurrection of Haitian institutions with an emphasis on health and education. The plan also sought, for the first time in Haiti's history, to guarantee a primary education to all Haiti's children. If such a plan is ever implemented it will be a godsend for the communities that Medishare works with in the Central Plateau.

That said, between the influx of refugees, the scourge and stigma of cholera and the shortened travel time created by the new national road, life on the Central Plateau has been forever changed. The splendid isolation that made Thomonde a "Shangri-La" is forever gone. The sense of community, in which everyone cared for each other, is threatened by an influx of new people, unfamiliar with rural life, and petty jealousies, as various factions compete for slow-to-arrive recovery dollars. It will take an enormous amount of energy on Medishare's part to prevent entropy and Baron Samedi from once again gaining the upper hand.

The fate of Medishare's critical care hospital is up in the air. Six months after the quake Medishare partnered with a small private hospital, to which it donated resources to improve its diagnostic and treatment capacity. Critical care is expensive, however, particularly if you are starting at ground zero. Two years of funding from the American Red Cross will soon run out and there is little prospect that these grants will be renewed. After the earthquake, the Medishare field hospital treated over 35,000 patients, performed over 3000 operations and fitted more than 2000 artificial limbs. In Haiti's time of need, no one can deny that the hospital was a *miwak*. Perhaps even more important than the thousands of lives that it saved, it gave hope to people who live on hope.